WHAT HAVE YOU GOT TO LOSE?

The Great Weight Debate
and How to Diet Successfully

SHELLEY BOVEY

GW00644995

First published by The Women's Press Ltd, 2002
A member of the Namara Group
34 Great Sutton Street, London EClV OLQ
www.the-womens-press.com

British Library Cataloguing-in-Publication Data
A catalogue record for this book is available from the British Library.

ISBN 0 7043 4715 6

Typeset by FiSH Books, London WC1
Printed and bound in Great Britain by CPD (Wales) Ltd, Ebbw Vale

To Gill Riggs for her courage and dignity

Contents

Acknowledgements

Huge thanks to all my friends for putting up with my neglect of them while I was writing this book and for still being there when I emerged from the tunnel. And to my family for just putting up with me!

Many people have helped flesh out this book (have you ever noticed how many metaphors there are to do with size and weight?!) You are too numerous to name, but I want you to know how much I appreciate your contributions.

However, there is one person who must be mentioned: Jill Welbourne has given me much of her time, patiently explaining the biochemistry of weight loss without once looking bored. Science never did come easily to me but when Jill explains it, it becomes positively accessible. Thanks, Jill, for constantly being there and for having your meals interrupted with such good grace.

And special thanks to Judith Durham.

Preface

This is the most difficult book I have written. Now, emerging from it, I feel as if I have undergone a thorough training in conflict resolution! I have tried to build a bridge between two apparently entrenched sides of the weight war: the one that believes that dieting is unnecessary, politically unacceptable and bad for you; and the other that holds that dieting is something that any woman over a size 16 has a moral obligation to undertake before qualifying for membership of the human race.

I find that the truth inhabits the middle ground, as truth always does. Absolutism – whatever it is about – is dangerous and leads to bigotry. Ideological inflexibility and intransigence do not take into account the fluctuating grey areas of human emotions, nor of individual doubts and ambivalences.

Like most large women I have suffered the blatant prejudice and discrimination that our society hands out to those of us who break the strict size rules. Until the eighties, there was no voice, no movement in Britain to speak for us, though America had been actively campaigning for size acceptance since the late sixties. When the movement began to gather momentum, when our politics began to be represented in mainstream media, we were too young and new a voice to compromise our stance by admitting to anything that might appear to weaken the cause – like the fact that many of us were not happy being fat.

The problem is that many, both in and outside the movement, would see a desire to be less fat as a contradiction of the political belief that prejudice and discrimination are an infringement of human rights. Somehow it is assumed that if you champion such a cause, you are perfectly at ease with your own status quo. Researching this book has shown me that is not necessarily the case.

There are many large women – I would dare say the majority – who have a passionate commitment to bringing about an end to prejudice, and yet who are not happy or comfortable in their own bodies. However sick and twisted society's rules may be, the fact is that we were meant to be social animals; it is not comfortable being 'different'. It is not just society, though. Our bodies were not designed to carry a great deal of weight; it can be physically inhibiting. For some, the quality of their lives is severely compromised by their size.

The first rule of size acceptance is that for many people weight loss is not an option. The second is that those who are truly unhappy with their size, for physical and/or psychological reasons, should be offered a way out. I believe that the only way to lose weight is to diet very, very slowly and to stay on a diet for life.

The purpose of this book is to show that it can be done and that those who, like me, choose to do it, are not betraying any cause. My commitment to the size acceptance movement remains the same. We have not as yet been an instrument for social change, but we must keep fighting.

I have already been criticised by those who believe that wanting to be less fat disqualifies me as a size-acceptance activist. To them I would just like to repeat something said to me long ago by a very wise old woman. 'Things are never "either/or",' she said. 'They are "both/and".'

That is the spirit in which I have written this book.

Shelley Bovey
Somerset
August 2001

Part One
The Great Weight Debate

Chapter One
Living in a World Gone Mad: Fads, Fashions, and Folly

On the 7 June 1999, a letter appeared in the *Daily Mail* entitled – in huge headlines – 'It's time we taxed the fat of the land'. The writer, one Helena Fishlock-Lomax, is the founder of the Size 8 Club, an organisation for women who say they suffer persecution because of their slenderness. (I am not writing this on 1 April.) Ms Fishlock-Lomax suggests that just as alcohol and nicotine are drugs and therefore heavily taxed to discourage indulgence, we should tax those who are 'overweight through their own fault'. She helpfully suggests a tax of £1 per day per BMI (Body Mass Index) unit above 25.

This tax would help to pay towards the treatment of obesity and its related diseases, she says, adding that Dawn French, who is, she claims, 'dangerously overweight' should be 'more responsible' (how?) and complaining that Calista Flockhart, star of *Ally McBeal*, and supermodel Kate Moss get a poor press as role models.

'Because of the greed and lack of control of unnecessarily overweight people, normal slim women are being bad-mouthed,' she writes, adding that 'of course' those who are overweight for genuine medical reasons would be excluded from this tax.

Without – for the moment – setting foot in the minefield which constitutes the health/weight argument, let me just redress the balance. While Ms Fishlock-Lomax points the finger at Dawn French and bemoans any criticism directed at Calista and Kate, I should point out that the health of the latter two has been evaluated by a reliable health professional and found wanting.

Catherine Collins, chief dietitian at St George's Hospital, South London, assessed several 'icons': women that most other women seem to want to look like. Kate and Calista, Jodie Kidd, Victoria Beckham and Julia Roberts were all found to have a BMI of below 18, giving rise to concern. Collins pronounced Kate Moss (BMI 15.7) 'very high risk and would be regarded as an eating disorder at our hospital'. Of Calista Flockhart (BMI 16.7) Collins said 'I would classify her as a borderline eating disorder case, possibly anorexic.'[1]

The point about this letter is that, although it is silly, there are deeper, more serious undertones. The proposed tax, for instance. A moderately overweight woman – say height 5″ 6′, weight 12 stone – has a BMI of 27. If she were to pay tax in Ms Fishlock-Lomax's suggested bracket, she would be paying £14 per week. A very overweight woman of the same height – let's say weighing 18 stone – would be paying £105 per week. And a seriously overweight one of 23 stone would be paying £189 per week.

This isn't about economics. This is about punishment. Clearly no one who hasn't won the rollover Lottery jackpot would be able to pay such taxes. And clearly the imposition of such a swingeing tax could never work. And why should it? Following this to its logical conclusion, we should treble the prices of cigarettes and alcohol – and levy on their consumers a *per diem* tax as well. We should tax those who indulge in sport; after all, they cost the NHS a fair old amount with their injuries and chronic sports-induced conditions. And as for dangerous sports like climbing or motor racing… well, need I go on?

This letter – and the formation of the Size 8 Club – is a symptom of the backlash against the relatively new size-acceptance movement in Britain. While I no more agree with 'skinny-bashing' than I do with verbally abusing the overweight, the claims that thin women are being discriminated against are tenuous to say the least. After all there are millions of women who would like to look like Helena Fishlock-Lomax and not one who would choose to look like me. But according to Fishlock-Lomax, 'Reasons to hate being a size 8' include 'Having shop assistants say "Aren't you lucky to be so slim?"' This is usually said as a compliment but when one has spend the whole afternoon trying on clothes that are labelled 8 but are huge, it makes me want to *scream*!!!!'[2] Not quite in the same league as being denied health care, college places, jobs and promotion – all of which rejections are frequently experienced by the overweight.

On the Size 8 Club website there are some examples of the sort of 'insults' thrown at thin women. These include 'Aren't you skinny – have you always been like that?' Fishlock-Lomax contends that people are rude to thin people 'in a way that would start a riot if used in reverse' and says that people would not make equally rude remarks to fatter people. She believes that due to political correctness, fatness is protected, even celebrated. 'People are frightened to say "large" is unhealthy', she claims. In a climate that vilifies the overweight even more than was the case five years ago I do have to question which part of the universe she has been inhabiting.

Sticks and Stones... But Words Do Hurt...

Since the publication ten years ago of my first book on size politics, *Being Fat Is Not a Sin*,[3] I have often been asked in interviews if I think that the climate is changing; if the national consciousness of the fat person's right to equal treatment in every arena of society has been raised; if the larger body is becoming more acceptable in aesthetic, media or fashion terms; and if the persecuted overweight, in common with other minority groups, are at least being treated more justly in the name of political correctness if nothing else. When I am asked these questions I don't jump in with a ready answer, for there are gaps between interviews and I need to consider the current signs of fat acceptance, if any. I am constantly reviewing the evidence, holding up a wet finger in the wind to see if it has changed in our favour. So far I have to admit that the weather is still bad out there and fat people remain out in the cold of prejudice, rejection and discrimination.

Any prevailing ethos is reflected primarily in verbal expression, written or spoken, considered or casual. Take the tone of this leader from the *Daily Telegraph*: ostensibly a piece about the politics of awarding points in the *Eurovision Song Contest*. This was the year the prize was won by Dana from Israel, who was neck and neck with the Maltese entrant. 'Not until the last vote did Dana, the Israeli transsexual, trounce the portly Maltese girl, Chiara, who sang so plumply of love', exclaims the leader writer. Nothing more than mild offensiveness there, though no one would take this hack for a size-acceptance activist. It is, after all, the sort of insulting, crass remark endured all the time by those of us with unpopular Body Mass Indices.

But what follows is breathtaking in its viciousness: 'Chiara's handicap of quadruple chins, Bunteresque fringe and an outfit the size of Grand Harbour, was finally washed aside by the cross-dresser vote.'[4]

In all probability this was written by a man. Most broadsheet leader writers are men. It is also a right-wing paper with the sort of arrogance that stomps all over the sensibilities of people it thinks don't deserve to *have* sensibilities – the undeserving fat, in this case. If only that were all it was: male, right-wing chauvinism. If only the size-acceptance movement had at least penetrated the hearts and minds of women, of the left-wing press and – of course – of feminists.

Fatness and Feminism

Where size acceptance is concerned, it isn't enough to be a paid-up feminist. You have to be a feminist who recognises injustice in *all* its forms. It's no good thinking that feminists will provide a haven for the fat though because left-wing feminists can be just as venomous as right-wing men. Or right-wing women.

Sadly, personal experience has shown me that, when it comes to weight, women are women's worst enemies. It is never men who suggest that I would look or feel 'so much better' if I lost weight. It is never men who say 'Should you be eating that?' It is women who feel the need to comment about another woman's weight before they comment on anything else about her. I find myself in total agreement with food writer Nigella Lawson, who wrote that 'the feminist perspective is a vexed one, for this is so pointedly a tyranny of the sisterhood. It's not men that women diet for, but the unforgiving gaze of other women.'[5]

Germaine Greer, for example, looked up to by so many feminists as an icon with almost regal status, seems to have a problem with fat women. In an otherwise thoughtful and thought-provoking *Guardian* piece about eating disorders, food abuse and marketing pressures, she hones her pen for the attack. She writes about watching a 'hugely obese' German woman 'snatch up the chocolate ice lollies her children had abandoned and literally push them one by one into her face. Under the table her vast thighs were moving spasmodically in a grotesque version of orgasm.'

What Greer is doing here is holding up a portrait of a woman who possibly has an eating disorder (though not necessarily) but she has painted the portrait in a way that will make the reader say 'Ugh.' The article is full of good information about anorexia, bulimia, dieting and the consumption of junk food but only when she refers to the obese do her personal prejudices show themselves. Again, this is about use of language, but because she is not as blatant as the *Telegraph* writer – not once does she actually *say* that she finds the fat German woman disgusting – her portrayal of the woman without overt insults conveys even more powerfully her distaste for fat people. Like many other fat-haters she couches her prejudice in a spurious concern for those with eating disorders. She also, perhaps surprisingly for one who is capable of showing great intelligence, resorts to the tired old stereotype about fat people stuffing their faces. Obese people, she claims, 'feed themselves junk on demand when no one they know can observe their obscene pleasure.'[6]

In a similar, though much more moderate piece, feminist writer Joan Smith looks at the polarisation between the 'fat is good' faction of the size-acceptance movement and the thorough condemnation of obesity by health professionals. She quotes from a recently published interview with Andrea Dworkin, which refers to the latter's collapse and subsequent hospitalisation with bronchitis, pneumonia and blood clots. According to Smith this 'graphically revealed the risks that she and other fat people are running'. On whose authority does she assert this? Anyone can get bronchitis, pneumonia and thromboses. The fact that thrombosis is claimed to be more common in fat people does not *ipso facto* mean that Andrea Dworkin's was caused by her size, but this kind of assumption is always made, usually without a shred of evidence.

While Smith is right to be alarmed at the fast-growing incidence of obesity in the western world, she too reveals her prejudices by the use of emotive language. She describes an aeroplane flight in which a man 'waddled up an aircraft aisle and subsided into the seat next to me. Rolls of flesh overflowed the armrest and I wondered how either of us would get out in an emergency.' Later Smith says we are constantly reminded of our insecurity by spiteful attacks in the media. Pots and kettles spring to mind, though Smith makes it clear that the 'we' refers to women. Are spiteful attacks on men okay then?

The trouble is that we expect feminists to be tolerant of those women who are perceived by society as deviant, and when they reveal the same prejudices as the rest we feel betrayed. When the

likes of Germaine Greer and Joan Smith show their distaste for
fatness it is somehow worse than Lynda Lee-Potter's full-on
attacks in the *Daily Mail*. Fat women assume they can depend on
feminists for support and validation but it is not so. The feminist
movement has not embraced size acceptance any more than the
rest of society, and we have to get used to that fact.

Eat, Eat, Eat – But Don't Get Fat

It is not the eating *behaviour* that is being condemned, even
though people speak with disgust about those who stuff their faces
with cream cakes or never stop eating. All those things would be
excusable if they did not result in fatness. You can, if you wish,
throw up your food (in private) without being considered a social
pariah. In fact you will be pitied; bulimia is a condition recognised
as being deserving of therapeutic treatment laced with
compassion. It is also, as more than one eating disorders expert
has pronounced, a 'fascinating' condition. Apparently.

There is a perverse kind of approval accorded to those who
can eat a lot and not put on weight, as though somehow the
large amount of food consumed and the lack of weight gain is a
kind of personal achievement. This suggests even more strongly
that eating behaviour is really of no consequence as long as you
don't get fat. As Llewellyn Louderback says in his brilliant book
Fat Power, 'It's one of those psychological, fool-the-eye things.
A fat person munching on a single stalk of celery looks
gluttonous, while a skinny person wolfing down a twelve-course
meal simply looks hungry.'[8] It's about perception, and about
what people see when they look at a fat person. What they think
they see is someone out of control, someone who is not
ashamed of excess, and this frightens them as body weight is the
only thing people feel is left to them to control in this
fragmented society.

As Helena Fishlock-Lomax demonstrates in her letter, it is
those who are perceived as 'fat through their own fault' who must
be punished. Being fat is a crime, a sin, in the eyes of the majority.
The kind of acceptance accorded to other minority groups is not
available for the fat. This is why the size-acceptance movement is
more important than ever because not only is the situation not
improving, it is getting worse.

Body Image and the Media

Where It All Began

I am old enough to remember the fifties, when a curvaceous size 14 was considered a desirable shape by men and women alike and the androgynous female body was not something to yearn for. In fact so worried were women that they might be too thin that there was an over-the-counter product called Wate-On. I remember my mother buying it. The fact that it has not existed for many years has little to do with trading standards legislation, though I see it is still going strong in Africa, where pharmacies do a roaring trade selling it to prospective brides trying to become fat.[9] The oft-quoted fact that Marilyn Monroe was a size 16 and the icon of her day serves as a benchmark for enviable body image of that time.

Then came Twiggy. The impact she made was because of her beauty: her huge eyes, perfect face and tiny, childlike body. We had not seen anything like it before and she set a new standard in modelling. She was young, she was vulnerable, and a great many people realised that they stood to make a lot of money from her. What is not mentioned is that Twiggy did nothing to achieve or maintain her size. 'I appear to be the epitome of the first skinny teenager,' she says in her autobiography *Twiggy in Black and White*.[10] 'But that is exactly what I was. A naturally skinny teenager.'

She describes the frenzy that followed the discovery that she actually ate like a normal human being. When the media found out that she had porridge for breakfast they even wanted pictures of her eating it. 'What I should have told them was that I really liked it with condensed milk,' she says.

Twiggy's memories of childhood revolve around food. Her mother was a wonderful cook with her own catering business. 'Mum's speciality was puddings: syrup sponge with custard, spotted dick. Just the thought of them makes me drool even now. Though nothing seemed to put on any weight.' Her mother would always come home from functions she'd catered loaded down with bags of goodies for her children.

Twiggy's unrestrained eating, though, earned admiration because she remained thin. 'I have never had to diet in my life,' she says. 'It's a question of metabolism. Until I had [my daughter]

I ate anything and everything. I'm glad I'm thinner rather than fatter. But it's not a question of choice. It's genetic. You only have to look at my sisters. We're like three peas in a pod. Thankfully I'm now about twenty-five pounds heavier than I was in 1965 when my bust (if you can call it that) was thirty-and-a-half inches and my hips thirty-two... The lumps on my chest only became breasts after I'd had Carly.'

Even though Twiggy was so tiny, the ultra-thin body as we know it today did not catch on in the sixties. By then the ideal was a size 12, and though the hourglass curves of the fifties were not so fashionable, neither was excessive thinness.

It was the eighties that brought about the biggest change. Along with Thatcherism, greed, excesses of every sort, conspicuous consumption and the emphasis on acquistion all formed the prevailing ethos. Appetites of all kinds were running wild; spirituality was defunct. Body control entered the arena as part of a new faux-religious ethic. Interviews with female celebrities were not complete without reference to body size. Women otherwise perceived as intelligent confessed to yearnings to be childsize. TV presenter Anne Robinson smoked to remain a size 10: 'I wouldn't smoke if I thought that when I stopped I wouldn't put on weight. I desperately battle to be a size 10 and I'm a natural size 12', and the actress Patricia Hodge bemoaned the iron control necessary to maintain her size 8 figure.[11] *Why?* Why did these mature women, acceptably slim by any standard, yearn and fight to be less than a 'normal' size?

A study has shown that winners of the Miss America contest have been getting thinner over the years.[12] Since Miss America began in the 1920s, the winners have become 12 per cent thinner and 2 per cent taller. By the eighties, their BMI had dropped below 18.5, which is the World Health Organisation's cut-off point for unhealthy undernourishment.

At the beginning of the eighties, people were just beginning to hear about a strange disease called anorexia. Bulimia put in an appearance a little later. By the end of the decade, both diseases were rampant and the effect of anorexia on teenage girls was a cause for national concern. The death rate was becoming alarming. If ever a time was right for size acceptance to gain a foothold, that time was then.

Size Does Matter (or so We Are Told)

Instead – and in spite of the toll taken by eating disorders – the search for the perfect thin body rages on apace. Alarmingly, women of size 10 – the 'perfect' size, we were told – are expressing unhappiness with their bodies. The *Daily Mail*, in its health section, carried out an interesting study of four women, all size 10. Every one of them was dissatisfied with her figure. The first complained she went 'straight down like a tree trunk' and, far from asking 'Does my bum look big in this?', she said she would like a larger bottom. She did not diet. Another, though, who hid herself away in baggy clothes, was 'really strict about what I eat. I just stick to salads and fish . . . But when my willpower fails me and I do eat something which I know is fattening, the guilt I feel is overwhelming.' The third member of this survey – tellingly demonstrating the change in the 'ideal' body over the last fifty years – said despairingly: 'From having a thin, fashionable figure I now look like a curvy fifties pop singer – not something I've ever aspired to.' So this woman watched her diet constantly, often skipping meals, even though at 5′ 7″ she weighed only eight stone. And the last one said that when she looked in the mirror she did not see 'a slim person. All I see is a disgusting, fat stomach.' Her mother, obviously remembering the time when women were allowed to be shaped like women and not boys, has told her that 'a round stomach is part of a woman's body'. But this young woman is not convinced. 'The state of my body plays on my mind all the time,' she said.[13]

Feminist writer Suzanne Moore, writing about the case of Samantha and Micheala Kendall, twin anorexics who starved to death, questions whether even this terrible condition is so much a disease as just an extreme version of conformity.

> I cannot regard them purely as freaks, completely apart from supposedly normal women. Instead I can see how like the rest of us they are. Sick as it is, they have achieved the goal that is presented to all women in the Western world nearly all of the time – the goal of slenderness. And not just slenderness – extreme thinness is the identity badge of today's 'real', happening woman.

'Culturally, anorexia and bulimia are perfect solutions,' observes Moore. 'They are entirely logical. A culture that tells us both to consume more and more and still be thin is an impossible one in which to live.'[14]

The award for tasteless remark of the age must go to the well-known female pop singer who expressed her envy of African famine victims. 'I know it's dreadful, that they're starving and all that. But I'd love to be that thin.' There you have current cultural values in a nutshell.

Even size 10 is now borderline unacceptable if you want to be where it's really swinging. Carol Vorderman, she of the much-publicised diet, is now very happy. She is a satisfied size 8.

But the 8s won't be flavour of the month for long; size 6 has made its pernicious way into the shops. In America, they've done away with all pretence of sizing clothes realistically – what is really chic is to be a 'perfect size 2'. Or, to go even better, a size 0. Yes, girls, in the States you can now officially cease to exist, sartorially speaking. I am reminded of Princess Diana, talking about her bulimia, saying she wanted 'to dissolve like an aspirin'. And I am quite baffled at Helena Fishlock-Lomax's assertion that the chief aim of the Size 8 Club is 'to make you feel less alone – it is not currently fashionable to be a size 6/8'.

Why are women so gullible when it comes to size and shape? Why do they not realise that a dress size is simply a label and a label can say anything a manufacturer wants it to? Dress sizes are no longer coded by a woman's measurements in the way they used to be. Before appearing to disappear became fashionable, a size 12 was a 34″ bust, 24″ waist and 36″ hips. And the magical size 8 was 30, 20, 32. Now honestly, how many women, especially mature women, actually measure 30″ round the chest and 32″ round their hips? I was delighted to hear the no-nonsense Esther Rantzen, who looks about the same size as Carol Vorderman, admitting to being a size 12.

A useful piece of research carried out by the Size 8 Club revealed that designer label size 8s vary from bust 32.5″, hips 34.5″ to a 'gigantic' bust 35″, hips 37″.[15] As Helena Fishlock-Lomax points out, these sizes are 'to fit' so the garment may actually be three inches larger than the stated measurements. What happens to women's brains when they buy clothes then? Are they really seduced so much by the idea of wearing a size 8 that they will go to the manufacturer that confers this Cinderella-type wish upon them? 'Buy this dress and you shall go to the ball as a size 8, even though in the cold light of morning you will remember that actually you have 38″ hips.' For those who were as puzzled as I was at the time, this explains why Vanessa Feltz allegedly metamorphosed into a hefty size 12. I myself am a size 20, but I have several garments which are size 18 and a bit baggy, and a size 16 dress which swamps me. It is so voluminous that a 14 would still be on the large side, so in that particular make I obviously need a 12! What nonsense!

There is a darker, contrary side to this resizing. Boutiques for very young people tend to deal in very skimpy clothes, as though fulfilling the expectation that their pubescent customers will be obediently dieting to look like the media representations they are supposed to be emulating. One mother angrily told me of her 15-year-old daughter's excursion to buy a top. She has a 36″ bust. And in that particular boutique the top that fitted her was labelled XL. What kind of message does that give a normal-sized teenager? I've seen these clothes myself when shopping with my daughters and have on occasion picked up a jumper I liked, thinking I could buy it because the label said XL. When I saw that it would obviously fit just half of me I laughed in derision. But then I'm not a deeply vulnerable teenager.

The Incredible Shrinking Women...

And then there is the parade of media role models: Calista Flockhart, Jennifer Aniston – who was thin but now, after following a faddy, high-protein diet, is even thinner – Courteney Cox, Portia de Rossi, Posh Spice. However much the Size 8 Club might protest that those who are 'naturally slender' are being discriminated against by being labelled anorexic, these particular icons have definitely lost weight since they hit the limelight – and they were thin to start with. Portia de Rossi, for example, admits to being 'caught up in the Hollywood paranoia about weight'. Jennifer Aniston lost 30 lbs to get the role of Rachel in *Friends*.

Refreshingly, Courtney Thorne-Smith of the vacuous *Ally McBeal* show has come clean and told the story of her own obsession with thinness.[17] It's a familiar tale in the media: a slim young woman is given a television role in which she feels fat next to her even thinner co-stars; she goes on a series of bizarre diets and becomes underweight, runs eight miles a day and feels 'exhausted and cranky'. In this case, though, intelligence prevailed, when Thorne-Smith started being named in articles about actresses who were becoming too thin. 'I'd been an advocate for health and fitness for a long time, so to be included in coverage about extremely thin actresses who damage young girls' self-esteem was a real eye-opener,' she says. 'I used to joke with my friends that I wanted to be a role model for being healthy, but that I wanted to be "really, really thin" while I was doing it. Suddenly I saw how unfunny that joke was.' The result was that Thorne-Smith started to eat properly and got her energy back. But the pressure she and her kind are under to be thin, thin, thin is revealed in an almost throwaway remark. 'I know some people might think I'm being overly demanding by asking to wear clothes I feel comfortable in, rather than forcing myself to fit into small clothes that are easy to find. But at the same time I feel proud that I've set my own standards. There will always be people who criticise – I can't win that fight, so my goal is to stop listening to them. After all, it's my own body I'm beating up, and why would I want to do that?' Thank God for one voice of sanity but it's not going to change the world, I'm afraid. It's not as though Thorne-Smith is even approaching any degree of overweight, not by any standard. She's just entering a plea to be allowed to have a normal body.

Vonda Shepard, the resident singer on the *Ally McBeal* show, is perfectly slim. 'Is there pressure on me to stay slim because I'm in *Ally McBeal*? Of course there is,' she cries. 'Calista is like a doll, she's tiny. I have never been fat but sometimes I look at myself on the show and I think I look enormous. I work out six days a week for at least an hour and a half at a time, because I know that it's part of my job to stay thin.'

Everyone in Hollywood is on the same diet of salad, steamed vegetables and a tiny bit of protein, says Shepard. No pasta, no bread, no salad dressing. Eating is a non-event. 'It's so boring. I hate it... The pressure never stops.'[18]

Someone who admits she has never been fat but who looks at herself and sees someone 'enormous' has obviously made a wrong connection somewhere. There is a proliferation of a new condition: 'body dysmorphic disorder'. This is a fancy Greek name meaning that you don't like your body and, if you are thin, you believe you are fat. It's a good way for stars to grab yet more publicity. First they are celebrated for their thinness (or castigated for being more than a size 10). Then having made their mark, they give confessional interviews which tell of their 'torment of insecurities' about their looks.

The actress Uma Thurman is one such 'sufferer'. Though fêted for her looks – in 2001 she was signed up as the new 'face' of Lancôme cosmetics – and possessed of a body so thin that she is described as an 'angular beauty...[whose] shoulder bones stick out and her trademark cheekbones seem sharper than ever', she apparently believes she is fat, thus earning herself a full page in the *Daily Mail*.[19]

I cannot sympathise with these women when fat people face abuse in one form or another every day of their lives. One thing needs to be understood: there is a world of difference between disliking your own body when all the external evidence assures you that you are beautiful and acceptable, and being less than comfortable in your skin because you are told at every opportunity that your fatness is ugly, reprehensible, unacceptable and a basic indicator of your flawed character. I am tired of here-today-gone-tomorrow stars bemoaning their looks when they have the sort of looks for which the majority of women would sign a Faustian pact.

...And Some Voluptuous Icons

So let's get one thing straight. Media representations of large women are not getting any better or fairer, give or take a few exceptions. I am not going to be curmudgeonly about this. I want to celebrate the exceptions. Pauline Quirke, for example, has been recognised for the very fine actress she is and though she gets a number of 'character' roles she has also played several parts requiring considerable depth: notably in the televisation of Minette Marrin's novel *The Sculptress* and in the popular and aptly named series *Real Women*. My only niggle about this is that her role in *The Sculptress* was that of a psychopathic murderer, and in *Real Women* she was the downtrodden, anxious one in an unsatisfactory marriage – though eventually she did get her man.

'I don't think about my size. Ever,' says Quirke. 'I've never considered myself to be a fat actress. I'm an actress who happens to be overweight.'[20]

Good woman. But I shall be even happier for her if she is allowed to play a strong role that doesn't pathologise her in any way; a role with status and authority, the sort of role given to Helen Mirren or Judi Dench.

It's not that large women are *not* represented on screen but, too often, if they are not pigeonholed in their comedian/agony aunt stereotypes, they are portrayed as deviant or just plain repellent. Lowri Turner, in an over-eager attempt to plead the case for her bigger sisters, drops us all in it when she offers Kathy Burke as an example. Claiming that she is one of film's 'most bankable stars', she enthuses that 'Kathy, an award-winning film actress, is still most famous for her role as the overweight, tracksuited Waynetta Slob in the Harry Enfield TV series'.[21] Quite.

I've sat over my keyboard for the last five minutes trying to think of other large role models, of other signs that we are being better represented in the media but my screen remained blank. Dawn French, of course; another wonderful actress and who doesn't love her in *The Vicar of Dibley*? But Dawn is one of those very few women who have made it in spite of their size, whose talent and personality have shone through so that she is forgiven for her fatness. That's the awful thing though. That there is something to be forgiven for in the first place but there is, believe me there is.

Actress Jade da Silva, size 16 and 5′ 7″, has had agents telling her she would have to lose weight before they would take her on. 'You do have to be thin to be successful. You might be a better actress, but the leading role will always go to a skinny person.' This was demonstrated in the casting of the film of *Bridget Jones's Diary*, based on Helen Fielding's lightweight but popular book about a thirty-something, calorie-counting Englishwoman. The role was given to Renée Zellweger, a Hollywood actress, whose first task was to put on a stone. So even when the *character* is required to be fatter, the actress employed in the first place must be thin – and then she has to gain weight. I suspect a clever publicity ploy here. Predictably, Zellweger's dismay at becoming a normal-sized woman was widely reported, as was her newly dieted figure once she'd made the film. It was one of those 'everybody's talking about it' events – so of course 'everybody ' went to see the film.

There are other exceptions. You can be an agony aunt like Denise Robertson or Claire Rayner, all earth mothery and comforting, with the stereotypical large bosom and broad shoulders on which the suffering may weep. You can be a comedian, like Jo Brand, as long as you are self-deprecating so that people can see that you are suitably apologetic for your size. You can make a huge name for yourself as a presenter like Jenni Murray – a *radio* presenter where your talent and personality and brilliant interviewing skills will be appreciated in full, as long as you can't be seen. Fortunately, Jenni Murray's exceptional work has been recognised and judged on its merit: she *is* allowed to appear on television.

Fat apologists also point to examples of what they see as mainstream media acceptance. They have cited Victoria Wood (who is no longer fat), Vanessa Feltz (of the much publicised six-stone weight loss) and the young actress, Lisa Riley, from *Emmerdale*. But this last was given a role that portrayed her as somewhat less than intelligent and her 'promotion' to presenting the puerile programme *You've Been Framed!* hardly struck a blow for fat women everywhere. When it comes to the States, the apologists trot out the tired and dated examples of Oprah Winfrey (who hired her own personal trainer and chef to help her lose weight and still put it back on) and Roseanne Barr (who had surgery to reduce her size).

Maggie Millar, an outstanding Australian actress best known in Britain for her role in *Prisoner: Cell Block H*, had the courage to leave the profession for many years in protest at the blatant sizeism and ageism she confronted. Now she runs workshops and seminars on body image, size acceptance and eating disorders. She is a natural performer and her message is mixed with readings and dramatisations that enthral her audiences. Beautiful, dignified and totally at home in her own skin, she has found a niche for her talent. Fortunately, television drama realised what it had lost.

Clarissa Dickson Wright and Jennifer Paterson, the much loved *Two Fat Ladies* of television cookery fame, did break the mould, there's no denying it. But they did so as much by their eccentric refusal to toe any conventional lines as by their size. With their almost anachronistic plummy voices and their disregard of correct televisual kitchen hygiene, they appealed to a nation rather too fed up with the wagging finger of the nanny state. On the whole viewers delighted in them, though there was a sizeable proportion of dour-faced doomsayers complaining about their liberal use of high-fat foods like butter and cream. They were a huge hit in the States, where a less purist ethos abounds and where they were able to accept Clarissa and Jennifer in the spirit in which they presented themselves.

Pop Stars and Other Singers

But if you're large you can't make it as a pop singer. Remember the fabulous and compulsive ITV series *Popstars* (January/February 2001), where a five-piece band was 'manufactured' from 3000 eager and talented young hopefuls? One of the most talented, with a stunning voice and a big personality, was Claire from Glasgow. She made it through several rounds but she was eliminated because she didn't have 'the right look'. As if they would ever put Claire in a pop band! She was a big young woman. She wasn't disappointed, though. She was totally realistic the whole way through, knowing that in spite of her considerable gifts, her weight meant that she didn't stand a chance.

This was more than proven when the band was finally chosen. The three female singers, Kym, Suzanne and Myleene, were all slim. But in one fly-on-the-wall programme Nigel Lythgoe, head of entertainment at London Weekend Television and the master-mind behind the series, confronted the clearly not overweight Kym and told her she needed help. 'You need to lose weight', he said, uncompromisingly. Kym, upset and obviously taken aback, asked for that piece to be cut from the programme. 'It's ******* out of order,' she said and left the room in tears. It was the first real confrontation of the series, but Lythgoe was unrepentant. 'Kym has taken it as a personal insult,' he said, as though there *was* another way to take it. 'If you're going to get up in front of the camera you have to worry about everything. You've got to look your best . . . this whole process of taking people and moulding them is the superficial side of the business. You have to look good. I don't know that many *fat* popstars.' Replaying that bit in slow motion, it was very clear that his lip curled in a sneer on the word fat.

Such was the extraordinary appeal of *Popstars* that it would have been an opportunity to go out on a limb, to dare to do something a bit different: to do in fact exactly what Lythgoe said was impossible and let one of the group be fat. I believe it could have worked. Millions and millions of viewers were rooting for that band before they'd even made their first record, because they felt as if they knew them. They'd watched them go through each round without being eliminated; they'd shared their euphoria when they were finally chosen. The viewers had bonded with the band and they would have done so just as much if one had been overweight, I am quite certain. I think Lythgoe and those with much invested in this were worried about how it would reflect on them if they selected someone who didn't have the 'right look'.

But in the sixties we had a superb and much-loved singer: Mama Cass, lead vocals of the immensely popular group The Mamas and the Papas. They immortalised 'California Dreaming', a song which has become a classic. Cass Elliot was a mountain of a woman in every sense, a huge body and a huge personality. She had style, she had sex appeal and she gave confidence to teenagers worried about their weight. Nancy Roberts, founder of the Spare Tyre Theatre Company and one of the early size-acceptance campaigners, said of Mama Cass: 'She was this wonderful sexy role model and inspiration who made it less of an incriminating burden to be fat.'[22]

Although outwardly the epitome of self-confidence, Cass was insecure about her weight and would go on bouts of semi-starvation which seriously compromised her health, hospitalising her on occasion. When the group broke up and she went solo, she felt the pressure to be thin even more acutely and went on ever more desperate, crazy diets. When she died of heart failure there was little doubt that the diets played more than a passing role in her death. She died alone and widely circulated reports that she choked to death on a ham sandwich had no foundation. 'It's been hard for my family with the sandwich rumour,' said her daughter, Owen Elliot, who was seven when her mother died. 'One last slap against the fat lady. People seem to think it's funny. What's so darn funny?'[23]

Then there was Rita Macneil in the late eighties and early nineties: a large woman with a haunting, bluesy voice. In her native Canada she had four double platinum albums and one of them knocked Madonna off the top of the Australian charts. She caused a storm in Japan and became Canada's biggest selling album artist. 'Rita who?' you are probably asking. She did come to Britain but she caused hardly a ripple. Sometimes this country doesn't know how to recognise quality.

It recognised Alison Moyet, though, another large singer. Moyet's image was of gutsiness and power, but she isn't Here and Now. She's been consigned to the past as far as the pop world is concerned.

The truth is that if asked to name large-sized women in the millennium-style pop business, the music industry would scratch its collective head and come up with Geri Halliwell (before she dieted) and Baby Spice (a size 10–12 when she should have been 6–8).

Even large opera singers are for the chop now. Deborah Voigt lost six stone after losing several roles because of her weight. Jane Eaglen, Britain's leading soprano, lost quality as well as weight when she shed seven stone. Her voice recovered when she put the weight back on. According to the dramatic soprano, Marie Hayward, producers now want an all-round performer who looks good and sings well enough, rather than a fat singer with an outstanding voice. The new slim breed of female opera singer often has to wear a hidden microphone in order to project her voice.

And women in high profile orchestras have been ordered to cover their arms because overweight arms are unsightly.

The Body Image Summit

In May 2000, the British Medical Association's Board of Science produced a report expressing grave concerns about the portrayal of unrealistically thin women in the media.[24] It claimed that women in the public eye often have half the body fat of an average healthy (non-fat) woman but that teenagers and young women are dieting in an attempt to emulate these role models.

Dr Vivienne Nathanson, head of professional services at the BMA, said that successful women are only seen to be attractive if they are thin. The report states that 'The degree of thinness exhibited by models chosen to promote products is both unachievable and also biologically inappropriate and provides unhelpful role models for young women. Female models are becoming thinner at a time when women are becoming heavier, and the gap between the ideal body shape and the reality is wider than ever.'

The BMA report also states that television producers and advertisers should review policy and practice when it comes to employing very thin women. The Independent Television Commission also has an obligation to review its advertising policy.

Chloe Cunningham of Cunningham Management in London, an agency which represents television presenters, has been concerned about unrealistic media images for many years.

> I get terribly fed up with producers saying a client of mine is overweight and being asked 'Could she lose a few pounds?' when she is absolutely not. It's getting to be a different race on television to normal life. It's disgraceful. Even people like Gaby Roslin and Carol Vorderman, who weren't fat, have felt the need to lose even more weight. Television has created a fake idea of what's normal . . . some women in prominent jobs are getting so vain they want to look like a skull. In real life they look ill.[25]

As that wonderful writer Nicci Gerrard mordantly speculated: 'If a Rip Van Winkle woke from a 50-year sleep today, and turned on the TV what would he think? He'd think maybe that he'd jump-cut forward to a time of plague or terrible famine; that some apocalyptic illness had ravaged the world. He would see famished-looking women with jutting collar bones and over-large eyes. If he went to a fashion show, he would see long-legged, fleshless, impossibly gorgeous and unnatural creatures on the catwalk.'[26]

The messages in the BMA report were reinforced in June 2000 by the Body Image Summit convened by Tessa Jowell, then Minister for Women. It all went horribly wrong, though the intentions were above reproach. It was announced at the Summit that the Broadcasting Standards Commission was to ask academics to monitor programmes to see how many women of average weight were portrayed. The aim was to stop the Ally McBeal figure becoming the norm, thus taking pressure off teenage girls to diet to unrealistic proportions.

The Tories fell on Tessa Jowell, claiming that the idea was political correctness gone mad. Ms Jowell stuck to her guns, asserting that there was ample evidence that the portrayal of thin women in the media caused women anxiety about their own weight. While the BSC said it would try to understand what influence, if any, broadcasting had on body image, it denied any suggestion that it would monitor the numbers of thin and fat women on television.

The Battle of the Glossies

Liz Jones, at the time editor of British *Marie Claire*, who spoke at the summit, decided to challenge the status quo. She produced an issue of the magazine with two covers: one with size-6 Pamela Anderson and the other with size-12 Sophie Dahl. She invited readers to choose between the two women: Sophie Dahl was the preferred model, suggesting that some readers of glossy magazines *do* want to see a more realistic image of womanhood.

The covers struck many chords. But Liz Jones was disappointed by the lack of backing from her peers. She wrote:

Newspapers, radio and TV stations were largely behind us. Our covers were in the national press for weeks, even making headlines in the New York *Post*. I had requests from universities here and abroad wanting to include our experiment in their college courses. Documentaries were made in America and Germany. The response from readers was unprecedented. However, the very people from whom I had expected the most support – my fellow female editors – were unanimous in their disapproval.[27]

Liz Jones had undertaken to bring together a group of magazine editors, designers and other professionals to act as a watchdog committee to monitor their own industry and to formulate a code of practice for self-regulation, whereby their publications would contain quotas of larger role models and the numbers of thin women appearing would be restricted.

The proposed campaign was widely reported, with such headlines as 'Magazines ban anorexic models'. But the press coverage had been premature. Not one other editor agreed to take part.

Instead most of them were hostile and aggressive. Jo Elvin, then editor of *New Woman*, accused *Marie Claire* of 'discriminating against thin women'... The day after the summit I received a fax signed by nearly all the other editors of women's magazines and some model agencies, stating that they would not be following any inititative to expand the types of women featured in their magazines... Alexandra Shulman, editor of *Vogue*, denounced the whole campaign as a promotional tool for *Marie Claire* and said that suggestions of an agreement to set up a self-regulatory body within the industry were 'totally out of order'... Fiona McIntosh, editor of *Elle*... accused me of 'betraying the editors' code'.[28]

A year after she began her campaign, Liz Jones resigned as editor of *Marie Claire*.

I reached the point where I had simply had enough of working in an industry that pretends to support women while it bombards them with impossible images of perfection day after day, undermining their self-confidence, their health and hard-earned cash... I could not have anticipated the extraordinarily hostile reaction from fellow editors and designers to my fairly innocuous suggestions. A year later I have come to realise the sheer terrorism of the fashion industry and accept that, alone, I cannot change things.[29]

Vogue had already been in trouble over its thin models. In 1996, the magazine was criticised by one of its advertisers, Omega Watches, for using anorexic-looking models. The complaint attracted press attention and subsequently a rumour began to spread that *Vogue* was planning a special issue featuring large, voluptuous women. That turned out to be rather far from the truth, but the June 1997 issue gave us a size 16 model, following a feature on beachwear which depicted excessively thin superwaifs. The idea for this came from photographer Nick Knight, who had discovered the 21-year-old Sara Morrison and who claimed that designers had to embrace the larger look if the portrayal of women in magazines was to change. 'When I was doing the shoot I felt we were breaking some taboos,' he said. 'It's a very positive image. She's supposed to look powerful. I didn't want to make her look freakish.'[30]

If nothing else it was a clever publicity ploy for *Vogue*; predictably the press was full of reports and features about the new large model. Journalists rang to ask if I thought this was the beginning of a new trend. I said no, it had happened before in other magazines and it had never caught on. It was, I said, tokenism; doing something different because of the splash it made. Besides, the magazines might use a size 16 model in one issue but would they use an 18 or a 20? I think some interviewers felt I was being negative but I'd seen it all before – it had come and it had gone. As Sara Morrison herself said prophetically at the time: 'There may be a bit of excitement for a week about it, then they go back to liking thin people.' QED.

Tokenism it was. *Vogue* editor Alexandra Shulman made it clear that real women – meaning a cross section of shapes and sizes – would not be appearing in her magazine. 'I wanted the pictures to be a kind of celebration of flesh but we're not about to use girls that are size 16. This is a one-off.'[31]

There appeared to be hope for the larger woman in the size 14–16 shape of model Sophie Dahl, who rose to prominence and gladdened the heart of the nation's 50 per cent of women who are size 16 or more. Tall and stately, she appeared to wear her size with pride and insouciance. But even 'small' larger women like Sophie Dahl have to cope with verbal attacks. 'While I appreciate Ms Dahl has a pretty face, I cannot help but wonder what she will look like in 10 years time if she is that large now!' wrote Helena Fishlock-Lomax of the Size 8 Club. 'I also wonder if Sophie Dahl is perceived as saying "stuff all the chocolate and chips you like and look like me, don't bother establishing healthy nutritional guidelines".'[32]

Dahl bowed to the inevitable pressure and lost weight. So did the actress Kate Winslet, who apologised for dieting but was afraid that if she didn't, she'd lose work. 'The urge to ally yourself with the forces of oppression is sickeningly seductive,' wrote Nigella Lawson. 'No intelligent woman seriously thinks she will be better if she's thinner.'[33]

What some editors said after the Body Image Summit, pouring scorn on the notion that their underweight models might be disastrously affecting the lives of teenage girls, was that you can't 'catch' anorexia; that it's a wider and deeper issue than it is a fashion or an aesthetic one.

True. But US researcher Aaron Lynch has discovered that certain behaviours *can* be catching. In his book *Thought Contagion*, he examines copycat behaviour and its relation to dieting. Thought contagions are 'the ideas that program for their own spreading in the human population much as a computer virus programs for its own spreading on the Internet. One of the most important areas of health affected by thought contagions is the area of eating disorders.'[34]

> The more dramatic a dieting behaviour – having only two carrots at lunch or taking an hour to eat half a bagel – the more it catches others' attention and causes them to try it. The most extreme over-exercising ideas also become more conspicuous, helping them to spread to others. Extreme versions of the 'skinny is beautiful' idea can spread around the office like an influenza virus, simply by catching more attention than ideas leading to a healthy weight that catch less attention by being more ordinary. The same effect also happens in the media, where the most unusual images are used to catch peole's attention for commercial purposes, regardless of whether they send healthy messages to the audience. Thus a model or actress who is shockingly thin or who looks like a heroin addict may catch people's gaze and hold it a little longer than does a model or actress who looks more normal. Since the purpose of most commercial media is to catch attention long enough to convey an advertising message, these models and actresses might bring in more revenue and thus advance in their careers, even if the images they convey are not particularly healthy to the viewers.[35]

The Marks and Spencer Campaign

Just after the doomed Body Image Summit it looked as though there was hope on the horizon. Marks and Spencer, the ailing high-street chain store, published the results of the biggest ever study of the female figure, which revealed that British women have become up to 20 per cent larger since the 1920s. The average waist is eight inches bigger, hips, six inches. In the 1920s as today, the desirable female size was 32-20-32; a size 8 in real terms. But our *skeletons* are now larger, making size 8 an unrealistic goal for most women.

The study, which took a year, used body-scanning technology to measure thousands of women. Everything from finger measurements to cup sizes was recorded and compared to measurements kept in the company's archives. It was official: women are growing. Size 16 is now average – and normal. It's a *healthy* size.

As a result, Marks and Spencer abandoned size-12 catwalk models in favour of size 14s, which is now its 'base' size. Although one in two women claim to be a size 12 or under, the study found that 60 per cent of British women are a size 14 or above. But surprise: modelling agencies could not provide Marks and Spencer with size-14 models. They did not have any on their books. The company employed an agency to work in-house, and they spent six months looking for size-14 women to model the new look.

Following this survey, Marks and Spencer launched a £20million advertising campaign which caused such a stir that the chain had more free publicity than it could ever have dreamed of. Television, radio and the printed media reported on it in such detail that you would have been forgiven for wondering if Marks and Spencer had gone into full-scale pornography in an attempt to salvage their dwindling fortunes. In their slightly bizarre television commercial, a woman runs up a hill, casting off her clothes as she goes. When she reaches the top, naked, she stands, arms out to the sun, and shouts 'I'm normal'. Only her back view can be seen. The explanation for the joyous cry is that she is a size 16 and quite happy about it, thank you. There is a suggestion of relief; as though she'd been in some way reprieved, rescued from the ignominy of outsize.

Which indeed was Marks and Spencer's point: that the 14+ woman should be able to come in from the cold and not feel in any way inferior to the size 10s and 12s. Following the Body Image Summit and other such initiatives, women were being offered the chance to escape from the tyranny of thinness. Maybe that was the place where the change could have begun.

But it didn't. And this is where it becomes apparent that it is women themselves who have rejected the move towards size acceptance.

A survey conducted by *Top Santé* magazine suggested that women are more obsessed with their body size than ever before. Of the 5000 respondents to the survey, 88 per cent felt that being plump was simply not attractive. Twenty-five per cent admitted to having taken slimming pills; 25 per cent had resorted to fasting and 60 per cent said they would have weight-loss surgery. More than 80 per cent felt inhibited by their body.[36]

Wendy Doyle of the British Dietetics Association stated that: 'This survey shows that perhaps Marks and Spencer has read it wrongly and that the average woman doesn't want to be a size 16.'[37]

Another survey, of 3000 25-year-olds, found that 68 per cent believed that their lives would improve immeasurably if they achieved what they considered to be the perfection of thinness; 78 per cent thought about their size and shape every single day; and 85 per cent felt that it was women who were their worst enemies, with their competitive criticisms of other women's size.[38] This last finding comes as no surprise for, as Suzanne Moore states, 'It is women who police each others' appearance.'[39]

Nigella Lawson felt that Marks and Spencer had missed the point. Knowing that size 16 is normal, she said, 'doesn't mean that size-16 women want to see themselves reflected in their own image. As any fashion magazine editor will tell you, their readers can write as many letters as they want demanding that more "normal-sized women" are featured in their pages, but the magazines they buy are the ones with the semi-starved waifs on the cover.'[40]

The early feminist Olive Schreiner had little patience with women. In 1911, she believed that they were obsessed with their face and clothes because they had no purpose other than to look good for boys. It would all change, she said, once women were allowed into the male world of work and had the power that would come from earning their own wage. The politics of appearance would melt away then and become a thing of the past. But now that women have achieved what Schreiner envisaged, nothing has changed. Not only do they not want to be fat, most don't even want to be a normal size.

Worryingly, this is not confined to the young; if it were, the chance of all body types being seen as acceptable would seem attainable. But women seem to have an ever-increasing fear of getting older. Carol Vorderman's new, childlike body was her fortieth birthday present to herself. And women with sound feminist credentials are not immune either. Nicci Gerrard, middle-aged, sharply intelligent and shamefacedly aware of her own gullibility wrote: 'I look at Calista Flockhart...and out loud I say "Oh God, she's horribly thin, she's ill, this is a nightmare"... and a small internal voice that I despise is whispering "She's much thinner than me. I want to be thin like that."'[41]

Older women like Joan Collins and Esther Rantzen are praised for looking 'great', ie for looking younger than their years. Nobody wants to look like Betty Boothroyd or Betty Driver (the very large *Coronation Street* actress who is in her eighties, still working, still as sharp as a tack with great energy and personality). Terrific women, neither of whom is glamorous in the way we have been socially engineered into evaluating glamour.

Why Size Acceptance Must Prevail

Size acceptance is one social change that the western world repudiates; the political integrity of such a movement is wilfully ignored or dismissed. Twenty years ago we could cite other cultures where fatness was not only acceptable, it was desirable. But now, increasingly, those cultures are turning to western values, adopting western diets and lifestyles and the people who once celebrated their large bodies are becoming less at home in them, juxtaposed as they are in white cultures with the sort of role models that this chapter has analysed. Worse, to congratulate or celebrate the large ethnic body is seen by some as a type of racism; for fatness is ever more associated with the negative qualities of sloth, gluttony, self-indulgence, lack of will power and lack of self-respect.

And therein lies the root of the resistance: fatness is not really a political or an aesthetic issue. It is seen as a moral issue. At a time when all other excesses – spending, sex, an increase in binge-drinking and recreational drug use – are increasingly socially acceptable, excess flesh is not. We have ditched all the once-held safe and containing beliefs about moderation in all things. So chaotic and anarchic is the result, where restraint is unheard of in most areas of our lives and considered unnecessary anyway, that there is a desperate attempt to retain some moral high ground. Where else to turn – since political correctness denies people all other avenues of overt oppression – but to the oppressed fat and to oppress them still more.

So where are we now? Is it true, as Joan Smith puts it, that 'Weight problems are part of a much larger anxiety about our place in the world, which means that learning to love obesity is as self-defeating as dieting to look like Kate Moss?' Am I being cynical and less than generous to society when I answer the question 'Are things getting better?' in the negative?[42]

I am not denying that there have been signs of *some* representation of *some* larger figures in the public arena. But it is not enough, nor is it consistent. Whenever there is an event celebrating size or a figurehead who appears to be gaining ground in society's acceptance of the larger body (be it only ever so slightly larger, like Kate Winslet), there is a backlash and any movement recedes again, like an outgoing tide. Many women confess to fearing fatness more than they fear death.

It is for this reason, this incoming and outgoing tide of size acceptance, that the movement is now more important than ever. In this ebb and flow, has there been any significant change, anything to suggest that the obsession with thinness, which at the turn of the millennium appeared more insane and unbalanced than ever before, might be on the wane? Might the tide be turning in favour of integrating and normalising all body sizes?

Not that, certainly. Women want to be thin with a sort of clawing desperation. Yet though the outlook looks bleak, though thinness prevails in a way it did not ten years ago, the size-acceptance movement in the western world continues to campaign for a better and more just society.

Chapter Two
Unlikely Bedfellows?: Reconciling Size Acceptance and Weight Loss

The State of the Movement

The size-acceptance or size-rights campaign is a human and civil rights movement dedicated to fighting the prejudice experienced by those who do not fit society's strict rules for body size. Founded in the United States in 1969 under the acronym NAAFA (the National Association to Aid Fat Americans), it did not really reach prominence or spread to other nations until the 1980s, when Britain, Europe and Australia became active in campaigning for equal treatment and acceptance of fat people. Even now the movement is relatively small; unlike similar human rights causes such as the battle against racism it has touched the hearts and minds of relatively few people. In every part of the world except a very few places in the USA, it is perfectly legal to discriminate against and abuse the overweight.

NAAFA (now called the National Association to Advance Fat Acceptance) has worked tirelessly to effect changes in the law and it is now illegal to discriminate against fat people in the City and County of San Francisco, in Washington DC, Santa Cruz in California and the state of Michigan. America has also seen law enforcement on the part of the Federal Trade Commission, which has come down hard on the weight-loss industry and forced it to regulate its claims.

Now, in the early part of the twenty-first century, the movement is slowly and steadily continuing to educate and inform. Sally Smith, one-time executive president of NAAFA and currently editor of *Big and Beautiful Woman* magazine, recognises that this is a slow process:

> I think when you look back over US civil rights movements, there's been a watershed event (Montgomery bus boycott, Stonewall, etc) that has mobilised people, as well as grassroots organisations. In order for the movement to succeed we need to

mobilise fat people. Look at those folks who protested at the World Bank and World Trade Organisation gatherings. I think that may be the new model for social change – the idea of small 'cells' of people who, within the cell may have a common interest but who may only have slightly overlapping interests with people in other cells. But if you get a critical mass of 'cells' working on the same issue, you'll effect social change. In order to be successful I think the size-acceptance movement has to restructure itself to accommodate changing times. If that happens, I think the movement can change the way fat people are perceived and treated.[1]

These 'cells' exist in Britain, Europe and Australia as well as Canada and North America, and they appear to have some power. The writings, conferences, exhibitions and individual stands of an activist nature attract attention and discussion. But although there is a great deal of media coverage of size issues, very often with quotes from size-acceptance representatives, the general population is not experiencing a sense of discomfort about a group – a large group – in society that suffers persecution and discrimination. Instead, as Chapter One demonstrates, there is a violent backlash against the very idea of size acceptance – as if white supremacy had risen to power to combat the move towards racial tolerance. Weightist equivalents of the National Front speak out without fear of censure; they have the force of most of society behind them.

The trouble is that relatively few non-fat people care enough about size acceptance to take up the cudgels. Sally Smith:

We need to learn how to cooperate and build alliances not only with large-sized people but with others who are sympathetic to our issues. We may not be successful in our initial attempts at organisation to change public policy. After all the National Association for the Advancement of Colored People was founded in 1909 and it took until 1964 to forge the first Civil Rights Act. That Act didn't come about until large numbers of people outside the Black community came on board because they recognised the importance of Advocacy, Education and Support for a group of people who had been systematically denied the benefits of our society.[2]

I think those of us who have worked in the movement for many years have had the edge of our first flush of optimism blunted. Some have dropped out and espoused other causes. The rewards are not easily come by. The die-hards will never give up, myself included. We *have* to fight for a more just world. But there are problems within the movement itself.

Like most movements for change, size acceptance has its factions and its unshakeable convictions. Like feminism, it is in danger of being divided against itself because of intolerance, in this case, around the issue of weight loss. We all know that diets don't work; that surgery is risky and can have appalling side-effects; and that drug treatment carries considerable risks. Those are some one of the reasons most activists oppose the idea of weight loss.

Size Acceptance in Britain

Diana Pollard, who founded the British organisation SIZE (the National Size Acceptance Movement) in 1996, remembers the early days of the movement as it assembled itself into what was then the Fat Women's Group. Though a convinced activist herself, she found their political convictions very difficult to work with:

I don't like exclusion politics. There was a lot of censorship, particularly around health issues. I disliked the censorship of articles for the newsletter, *Fat News* – articles that were to do with fat-related illnesses. There were women who wanted to discuss what it was like being a fat woman with diabetes or heart disease but this was censored. It was considered by a politically correct controlling element within the group to be making a negative response about fatness and so censored out.

On the one hand the group was uncompromisingly against all forms of weight loss but on the other hand it was unwelcoming to very large women because they were the ones likely to have negative personal experiences about being fat that go beyond discrimination, in that they had outgrown them-selves and their bodies were troubling them. Even if there were no discrimination, these women would still be in personal difficulty about being fat. And I'm not talking about a personal aesthetic, I'm actually talking about difficulties arising from one's size: pain, discomfort and unwellness.

So I didn't believe that this was the way forward for size acceptance in Britain. I believed we needed something with a far broader base, something that would put it out there as a human rights issue that could be accessible to everyone irrespective of their views about the rights and wrongs of fatness. I wanted to make a shift from the idea that fat is bad or fat is good: the glad-to-be-fat ethos, to move away from that and say the issue here is discrimination and discrimination is *always* wrong; it's damaging to society. I saw the movement as being inclusive for men as well as for women, and for anyone who supported size acceptance, not just fat people. I wanted to be part of an anti-censorship organisation where there would be no taboo topics; one where a person could be comfortable about being honest about how they felt about being fat, not to be afraid to say if they wanted to be slimmer or try another diet. My personal mantra has always been 'Freedom to be the person you are'.

I'm not interested in existing in a fat ghetto. The work I do is part of my overall philosophy. Some people find freedom very frightening. They find 'thou shalt nots' much easier to cope with – thou shalt not diet, support men, talk about sex, talk about illness, mention any difficulties at all about being fat. And the less tolerant that society is as a whole of fat people, and the harder the media come down on fat people the more this ghetto strengthens. The more insecure some fat activists get, the more rigid they become about rules.

For some years I have been uneasily aware of the factions within the movement. A movement for social and political change initially emerges as a minority group in society, therefore those within it can feel threatened, not only by wider society but by non-conformtiy within the ranks. Cohesion is of great importance but cohesion does not always mean agreement on the issues being addressed.

Size Acceptance and Weight Loss

I have written much about the pain and degradation of social prejudice and discrimination.[3] But I have been made aware over and over again of another type of pain: that of people whose size makes them so unhappy or feel so disabled that they retreat from mainstream life. These are usually very large people, not the size 18s or 20s but the 'super sizes'. No one should be that oppressed and the acceptance movement will continue to fight that oppression.

But we have to deal in reality: for physical and/or psychological reasons, some people are existing in bodies that are too big for them and it is more than they can bear. The purpose of this book is to try to offer a way through that: not based on the size-acceptance paradigm, nor on that of the thin-espousing society in which we live, but on the needs of the individual, who can feel very isolated.

When you are fat, you cannot help but be aware, most of the time, that you are different. That you don't fit, literally and metaphorically. That however much people may like, love or admire you, most of them would prefer you to be thin and that, wrong though it is, you offend most of society simply by existing. You are conscious of others' reactions to you, you imagine their thoughts (she'd be quite pretty if she weren't so *fat*, how could she let herself get like that, why doesn't she do something about it, etc, etc). If you deviate from the collective perception of what is aesthetically pleasing, you cannot help but be self-conscious – whether you've got a wart on the end of your nose or you weigh several stone more than most people. Of course, you can develop a compensating strength of character to mitigate the slings and arrows of condemnation but it is painful; the idea of self-love at all costs comes dangerously close to another tyranny: that of spiritual correctness.

A dear friend, with whom I have worked in the movement for years, and whom I had thought to be physically and emotionally at peace with her very large body, spoke to me one day of her weariness, using a powerful metaphor. Her house, she said, was suffering from overloading due to the piles of books she kept upstairs. She called in a structural engineer for an opinion. He said that the weight of the books was too great for the framework of the house. A lot of the books would have to go because the house was at risk of collapse. The house, she said, was her body, her skeleton. The books were her fat. Some books – some fat – would be fine. Just not as many, not as much as she and the house were carrying.

It takes a very stable and well-established sense of self-esteem to live happily in a society that hates you, or in a body that hinders you. Jane Goddard Carter is one such woman; I include her here because what she says is a celebration:

> Showing confidence in inhabiting the big, fat body is rare. Being confident in our size requires more energy and bravery than many people can muster. When we have that confidence we shine. We shine more brightly than any digitally enhanced, gaunt, pubescent coathanger who may gaze at us from every billboard or magazine page. When we arrive, we arrive big time. We can be loud, shy or just plain ordinary, but we are there, like it or not. So why not be as big as we are? Why live in a perpetual state of apology? I enjoy being big. I will not despise parts of me that wobble, crease or fold, just because I am told to. I will show my strength, my substance.[4]

Lee Kennedy, a leading – and brightly shining – light in the movement is one of the most talented women I know. She is an artist, a cartoonist whose work has power and wit and pathos. She loves opera and has a phenomenal knowledge of it. She is feisty, intelligent, funny and quick. But her lack of self-confidence led her into a mind-numbing job as a switchboard operator and a life only half-lived:

> I have been involved in size-acceptance groups for many years. It shames me to admit my real feelings about being fat because it shouldn't have to be like this. I feel a weakling and a traitor, but everything I have said is my truth. I admire and envy those fat women who are honestly able to build up enough self-esteem to put a finger up to the clucking, chastising, abuse-bellowing world. I believe in their goals but I can't see any hope of these coming to fruition the way things are going now. Appearance, and conforming to the 'right' look, seem to become more and more important all the time, instead of dying out. Women are still cursed with trying to live up to ridiculous, arbitrary ideals of appearance, and now men too must starve, work out, preen with the right products, invest in repeated cosmetic surgery (and don't think I wouldn't, if I had any money) – to be accepted, to get anywhere in life. Everyone's a product. As a middle-aged fat woman, of the

unbubbly variety, I'm an Edsel, a Strand ciggie, a great wodge of Lymeswold...

The politics of size acceptance should not be incompatible with the desire to lose weight. It is bad enough living in a fascist society that states that we are inferior because we are fat. But there is an intransigence in the 'fat and proud' camp in the movement which imposes another kind of fascism, that which suggests that anyone who does not accept their fatness is treacherous. This does not take account of the psychological pain experienced by those people whose lives have been so adversely affected by physical problems or by stigmatisation that they do not have the personal strength and conviction to be proud in their fatness.

Size acceptance must be at the top of the political agenda: a vital issue ranking alongside racial, sexual and all other forms of discrimination against those who differ from the white, hetero-sexual, Protestant model – largest permissible size for women being 16. But the movement has to acknowledge the validity of the feelings of those it is fighting for; among them are the thousands of men and women whose lives would be immeasurably improved if they could lose weight. Size acceptance should not mean you have to be fat and happy or fat and proud. I will not accept the imposition of self-love and self-acceptance as a condition of membership to the movement; nor can I accept that the contribution of those who want to, or do lose weight (whether 'successfully' or not) is less valid than that of those who choose to stay the size they are.

Because of the counter-pressure from the movement, Diana Pollard feels that SIZE may be out of step with other activist organisations because of its policy on weight loss.

SIZE gets mostly negative criticism as an organisation. We are mentioned with scorn in the media. Difficulties with other branches of the size-acceptance movement arise from our anti-censorship policy and our inclusion politics. There are always factions present in any movement.

There is very little positive to say about [weight loss]. Most diets end in failure. It's about changing what you eat, not eating less. There are people in SIZE who are dieting and they are experienced in the difficulties of permanent weight loss. They don't use drug therapy or VLCDs [very low calorie diets]. They aim for a very slow loss, building in activities. SIZE will support those who want to lose weight, but not if [those people] are bullied into it. Sometimes they need the support to stay as they are. When someone wants to lose weight for themselves we give them as much information and support as possible. We encourage them to change the type of food they are eating and increase their activity. We point them in the direction of a therapist for problems with overeating. SIZE is not about making personal decisions about people's lives. Some people do have to have another go at weight loss. They say they don't like being this size. The thing I like best about SIZE is its diversity.

How we feel about ourselves is complex. It's hard work to try and love our own bodies because every day we are bombarded with information telling us we're not good enough in diverse ways. It's possible to know where it comes from but not to be able to love yourself. It's an individual's right to change their position. People who join SIZE will have gained and lost weight several times over and deserve great compassion and support, not to be told they're a traitor. Wherever else they may be rejected, there is always a place for them here.

How could I hold my head up and say I'm antidiscrimination if I discriminate against someone who wants to lose weight? There has got to be a safe space for everyone.

NAAFA has a policy against weight loss based on its failure rate, but Frances White, a former president, wants to emphasise that those who attempt to lose weight should not feel that they are outside the fold:

Many NAAFAns have had weight-loss surgery because they couldn't deal with the pressure from society, employers, family and their doctors. Many of them drop out of NAAFA at a very critical time when they really need the social support NAAFA can provide. They drop out because they believe they will be hated by fellow NAAFAns. They drop out because the surgery doesn't work and they are embarrassed . . . We are here to fight for the rights of people of all sizes of large. Just because you have changed your body for now doesn't mean you are as thin as society wants you to be, doesn't mean you might not be large again.

Frances also raises the point that weight loss does not necessarily make you thin. A very large person can lose 6, 8, even 10 stone and still be fat.

The mid-size fat person suffers a lot of bias as well as a super-sized person. The bias may take different forms but bias-caused pain is just as painful. We understand this better when we look at the bias suffered by African-Americans. There is less prejudice against light-skinned Black people than against dark-skinned Black people. But the discrimination is very real no matter what 'tone' you are.

Diana Pollard believes that this safety to be ourselves and to state our individual needs is vital for the future of the movement.

I don't believe that it's outside forces that make an impression. I think [the movement] has the capacity to kill itself by its own intolerance. If I have a goal at all it's to try to create a climate where people can be honest. I think our magazine *Freesize* has demonstrated this. Outside of SIZE I don't think that environment exists. We're living in an increasingly hostile society. Things are getting much harder for fat people and I think it's going to get worse.

The intolerance in the movement, and the intransigence about weight loss doesn't help. I would like to see an end to Thou Shalt Not. We need more acceptance of differences within the movement. We have a common denominator: we are all shapes and sizes of large and as a result of that we experience discrimination. [We need to] accept that our common goal is to challenge that discrimination. There's no future if we attempt to police one another, to make rules about how people must be when they are fat. I think we need to challenge the idea of living by these rules. They're being made all the time by the government, by society, by the medical profession – there's no place for them in size acceptance.

A Word About Language

This seems to be the place to address the difficulty with weight-related language and the further frictions this causes within the movement.

The word claimed by the movement is 'fat'. It is a word I have immense personal difficulty with. I hate being called fat. I shrink from calling other people fat (though I try to do so when I know it is a word they feel proud to own). But just as I respect others' desire to use the word 'fat', so I object to being coerced into using it because it is now politically correct.

My first book was initially called *Being Fat Is Not a Sin*. It was not my title and I did not like it. I did not demur, though, because the publisher felt it was a good, right-on title. It certainly said what the book was about; unlike most non-fiction books it did not even have a subtitle. But I was uncomfortable with it. When non-fat people asked about my work I avoided naming my book. Although I thought this was cowardly behaviour I could not help the way I felt.

For me, being called fat is like a black woman being called a nigger. I find it painful. It is redolent with insults, put-downs and bad childhood memories. So I use it sparingly. What is more, I have had letters from readers who also found the title difficult and shied away from asking for it in bookshops. Surely people's sensitivities should not be sacrificed to the Cause?

Charlotte Cooper, a prominent British size-rights activist and author of *Fat and Proud*, condemned the title change of my book to *The Forbidden Body: Why Being Fat Is Not a Sin*. 'Bovey has disowned those of us who can and do use "fat" to describe ourselves and to inform our politics,' she writes, even while adding that she empathises with my discomfort. Cooper quotes me as saying 'Fat activists will not approve of my evasive behaviour and I apologise to them, but being fat is so painful, such a sensitive issue for so many, that I believe we must keep that in mind at all times,' but then goes on to say that the name change is a 'retrograde step, like jumping back into the closet'.[5]

This sort of compulsion is what makes me uncomfortable about the fat rights movement. Cooper says, with regard to my decision, that she feels that 'it is wrong to deny such a central aspect of my life.' Quite. But I regard it as disingenuous to see my self-confessed ambivalence as a denial of *her* truth. It's like saying 'Unless you have good self-esteem I can't either.'

It is painful when people who long for something as vital to humankind as size acceptance cannot agree. My close friend the actress Maggie Millar is one of the most prominent movers in the Australian arm of the movement. The writing of this book is raising questions for both of us, though we know our friendship is strong enough to survive and grow through them. For Maggie, the language of weight is as sensitive as it is for me but we are sensitive over different words. Her words of choice are: large, tubby, round, generous, sturdy, big, plump, heavy, Rubenesque, gargantuan, imposing, fat, sensuous, curvaceous, voluptuous, stout, chubby and, plumptious. I like all of these except 'tubby' and, of course, 'fat'.

But Maggie abhors 'overweight' and 'obese', calling them 'value-laden, judgemental, unscientific, prejudicial and counter-productive. They are words which wound, shame and induce guilt in the very people health professionals purport to help.'[6]

You see, this is difficult. I absolutely agree with her about 'obese'. It is a vile, greasy, onomatopoeic word. I have cringed when I have seen doctors' letters or case notes about me and seen myself described as 'grossly obese', 'morbidly obese', and 'obese +++'. But if a doctor is going to insult me when I walk into a consulting room, it hurts less if he says 'You're overweight' than if he says 'You're fat.'

In this book, there will be no consistency in the way I describe those of us who weigh more than society or the charts say we should. I will use the word 'fat', but I will also use 'large' and 'overweight'. Although I agree with Maggie when she says indignantly 'Over *whose* weight?', I shall use it for convenience, simply because we all know to what it refers. I shall occasionally use 'obese' and 'obesity' in terms of clinical practice or evaluation, not as chosen descriptive words. And I apologise to anyone who is offended by my choice of language.

Shock, Horror – Activist Uses the D Word!
I will also say now that I shall use the verb 'to diet', meaning to adopt a reduced- (though never low-) calorie way of eating, and the noun 'diet', meaning a form of eating which leads to (slow)

weight loss. This is to avoid the ambiguity of such phrases as 'eating healthily' when used in the context of losing weight. Healthy eating maximises health; it does not lead to weight loss.

I use the word 'diet' deliberately. The word has been discredited because of its poor track record of success but just as size-acceptance activists have reclaimed the word 'fat' in order to remove its negative and destructive connotations, so I am reclaiming 'diet'. If you want to lose weight you will have to go on some sort of diet, ie you will have to restrict your calorie intake. While you *can* lose weight by increasing energy (calorie) expenditure through exercise, this rarely results in permanent loss.

To diet to lose weight is not a bad thing; it is the type of diet you employ that is the crucial factor for health and success. This is a time for calling a spade a spade; it is very definitely not a gardening implement and 'eating healthily' will not make you thinner.

So, while I feel the word 'diet' is admissible, anything that qualifies the word (in reference to weight loss) will be a temporary measure with built-in failure. So anything that calls itself the 'something' diet (grapefruit, cabbage, blood group, chocolate addict's, etc) will not lead to a permanent change. Dieting means eating normally, though with fewer calories than are needed to maintain a stable weight.

Daring to Speak Out

I had always believed in size-acceptance politics; in fact an article I wrote for a women's magazine in 1988 was entitled 'Being Fat Is Not a Sin: A Plea for an End to Prejudice'. It was the first such piece to appear in a mainstream publication and paved the way for the first British book on the subject.

However, I was not happy with my supersized body. Years later, by which time SIZE had come into being, Diana asked me to contribute to *Freesize*. I discussed with her my growing feelings of isolation, believing that not wanting to be as fat as I was would not be acceptable in a movement magazine. Far from it; Diana encouraged me to write what I felt. Her motto: freedom to be the person you are includes the freedom *not* to love my size. The article appears below, edited to avoid repetition.

I would like to pose a question which some may find provocative or even offensive, but it needs asking: what is good about being fat? I don't mean three or four stone above the 'ideal' weight for height, I don't mean a size 18, 20 or even 22. I am talking about being supersized, outsize, very fat. I don't need to define it further, we all know who we are, though I should say that this is not meant to be divisive. Anyone of any weight may feel restricted by their body. But studies have repeatedly shown that the longest life and the best health are enjoyed by those who are about 30 per cent heavier than they are told they should be for their height. These people may have a BMI that goes into the red, they may be discriminated against by society, but they have not outgrown their skin.

I use that rather curious image because it is what I feel about my own body: that I have gone beyond some physical boundary. Not one set by insurance company weight tables, nor doctors, nor women's magazines, but one which I recognise from within, from the place where my body speaks to me.

I don't know when I crossed that boundary. Of course it was gradual. At some point in the last seven years or so I became conscious of having 'grown out of my skin'. I was too big, physically too big, for me. I weighed $19^1/_2$ stone.

It should go without saying that provision must be made for large people in society. Of course we should be able to get good clothes easily, we should be able to fit comfortably into all seats, we should not have the humiliation of having to pay double on an aeroplane as some very large people do. That is part of what the size-acceptance movement is campaigning for. The reality, though, is that as yet it has not happened and it will be a long time before society fully expands to accommodate us rather than trying to squeeze us out. This is the reality that the very fat have to live with. And it does not feel good.

Recently I went for a weekend to Centre Parcs with my family. As I have ME I could not join in with the vigorous physical pursuits on offer there. Instead, I decided to treat myself to a massage. Treatments of all kinds took place in an attractive building with a spa pool and a lounge in which to relax, have drinks and look through big picture windows to a stunning view. At reception I was handed a white, soft, warm towelling robe, size L, and asked to undress and put it on. It would not meet over my breasts and stomach. I walked through to the treatment rooms, holding it awkwardly and trying to cover my nakedness with my other hand. To my horror there were men as well as women sitting around relaxing in white robes as I walked past. I did not enjoy the massage, I was too tense.

During our stay at Centre Parcs, my family decided the best thing would be to borrow a wheelchair so they could take me around with them. I thought it a good idea until I realised how difficult it was for my husband to push me. Somehow I had thought that weight would not be a problem with wheelpower but he, a fit man, was breathless very quickly. And there was the time my daughter, a fitness instructor, just could not manage to push me up a slope, and strangers stopped and offered to lend their weight. I could not help feeling a burden, literally. I have to say it was a humiliating experience, not being in a wheelchair *per se*, but being too heavy for my family to push me around with ease.

My illness was not caused by being fat but it cannot help but be exacerbated by it. ME means that your muscles, joints and limbs do not function properly. Dragging a heavy body around when energy levels are reduced to a fraction of normality is excruciating.

That there are health problems at high weights is irrefutable; to deny this would be burying our heads in the sand. Joints suffer. There is an increased risk of certain diseases. A 25-stone friend, paralysed since babyhood, a champion of the fat rights movement and a fierce opponent of dieting and surgical intervention, has now had a high-risk operation to make her stomach a fraction of its normal size. No one would help her with her addictive eating disorder and now, with sleep apnoea and congestive heart failure, she sees no alternative. Her life is at risk. And if this makes you angry, if you think she should not have chosen this path, what would *you* suggest she should do?

I admit I would like to lose weight. Not to become thin – that is not me. I would like to get back to my agile 12^1/$_2$ stone, though maybe plus a bit extra because it is normal to get bigger in middle age. For some bizarre reason, though, if I ever say this to friends they are horrified. 'You couldn't lose weight,' they cry. 'You'd be betraying the cause.'

What do they mean? What is the cause? To me, it's about the solidarity of fat people against a hostile society. It's about getting a fair deal and putting an end to the fascist and corrosive prejudice we endure. It's about equal opportunities and being able to belong, and it's about the giving and receiving of support to and from each other. It doesn't mean maintaining a high weight, though there is often little choice about that.

As I write this I find myself becoming angry with those who insist we must celebrate our fat bodies. The truth is that beyond a certain weight, they let us down. It is futile to protest that this is not so. I believe in dealing in reality, and for me it is more honest to celebrate our achievements and ourselves and our courage if we acknowledge that they are tempered with emotional and physical pain, embarrassment, humiliation and tears. After all, without these there would be no need for courage. There may be those who truly enjoy being very fat and, if so, I salute them. But I know there are a great many, the majority in fact, who do not.

Being fat is never a sin. It is never anybody's fault. But it can be disabling in many senses and I believe it's essential that we don't deny or gloss over that.[7]

Freesize magazine and I received a great deal of mail in response to that piece. Many of the letters were cries from the heart, from women who had wanted to admit to the kind of things I was owning up to but who had been afraid to do so. But there was anger too, which I had expected, from women who believed me to be a traitor.

One letter made me feel that my instinct in writing the way I did had been right, though it was a scary thing to do.

Thank you for writing as you did. I think your article may be a turning point in the ideology of fat acceptance. You are brave to have written it because there are those who will call you a traitor and tear you to shreds. But what you say is common sense. If we campaign for the right to be the size we are, then that must include the right to lose weight if and when we choose to do so

– as long as it is for us and not because society says we must. I can relate to your experience: I too am fit at 16 stone, but when I hit 17 I can't run for a bus or climb stairs without getting breathless or even do up my shoelaces. Whatever weight I choose to be I am medically obese and a social pariah but I am acceptable to me and I am comfortable. If other size–acceptance activists accuse you of betraying their cause then they are oppressing you just as much as society oppresses all of us who are fat. Thank you for confronting this.

Being happy in our bodies is, in the end, not about ideology. When we fight for gay rights it does not mean we want to be gay or would be comfortable being gay. If asserting the right to be fat is controversial in mainstream society, then I propose to introduce a counter-controversy; I want to assert the right to lose weight for all who wish to try and do so.

It is all a question of identity.

Chapter Three
A Question of Identity

In a perfect world nobody would be defined by their looks; there would be no competition or comparisons. In such a world, intelligence, personality, achievement, ability, humour, kindness and compassion would not only count more, they would count first. Media stars would not fill newspaper pages with their insecurities about being a size 10 when they would rather be size 8 or 6; glossy magazines would not upset the equilibrium of pubescent girls already trying to cope with the storms and changes of incipient adulthood, because there would be no place for these magazines. Being good enough would not depend on *looking* good enough so we would all start on a level playing field.

Anthropology and Culture

But that is a fantasy, one that I cannot see coming to pass. There are suggestions that our preoccupation with appearance is deeper and more primitive than we may think. It is evident in the animal kingdom, though strangely reversed: there the males flaunt the brightest plumage in order to attract the females who, on the whole, are dowdy and dull looking. This serious business of having what it takes to keep the species going apparently applies to human beings too; recent research claims that beautiful faces are symmetrical ones and these tend to belong to those with the most chance of longevity. It has even been suggested that obesity is repellent in society because the obese have shorter lives and therefore are less likely to be around to breed, though I think this piece of information is another weapon in the fattists' armoury rather than genuine scientific research.

At this stage of human evolution the biological imperative to reproduce is no longer dependent on mere appearance. Where size is concerned, even the anthropological differences and the formerly diverse markers of identity are merging so that cultures which once took pride in large bodies have been contaminated by the western preference for thinness. The degree of conformity in all aspects of appearance is alarming. Rebellion in the form of creating a deliberately separate visual and aesthetic identity from mainstream society seems to be on the wane. In the fifties there were beatniks, in the sixties, hippies, the seventies and eighties gave us the glorious anarchy of punk but the end of the last century saw a uniformity that is eerily synchronous with the moves towards cloning. Never has fatness been so unfashionable; never has the pressure to be thin been more insistent.

There is a powerful Canadian film called *The Famine Within*[1] that brings home the message that most women's identity is dependent on their body size with almost shocking force. In the film, women of all weights and ages talk about what size means to them. An anorexic woman, fully aware of her own predicament, nevertheless states: 'I'd rather die than be fat'. She may get her wish: around 15 per cent of anorexics do die.[2]

A teenage girl in the film, when asked what fatness connotes for her, replies: 'Fat and sloppiness, and...almost dirtiness; someone who can't take control of their life; someone who's just so washed up that they can't take control of something so simple as their weight, they can't hold it back. Someone with no will power or no determination is someone who's fat.' And another woman, when asked about her image of perfection, says: 'I think the ideal is a woman who is about 5' 10" or 5' 11" or 6', about 115–120 lbs, wearing a size 4, or a size 6 – tops – and just drop-dead gorgeous.'

These women are demonstrating their fervent and almost literal belief in the phrase 'you are what you eat'. Their sense of 'I-ness' comes from what size 'I' is. All things follow on from that.

'Such is the power of the visual media in our lives that they can actually determine our sense of reality even if it means overriding our direct experience. Thin is normal and everything else is an aberration.'[3]

I saw someone on television recently who I thought was 'drop-dead gorgeous': the American actress Camryn Manheim. She's the woman who, on receiving an Emmy for her work in the popular US legal series *The Practice*, joyfully raised the statuette in the air and shouted 'This is for all the fat girls!'

Fat, Proud and Defiant

Camryn Manheim is tall, with a fall of waist-length, straight shiny brown hair and a beautiful face. She has dignity, elegance, grace and presence. She is very fat and she wears her size with pride. Of all the professions that draw attention to your size and other physical 'failings', acting ranks among the highest. Like all fat actresses, Manheim found it hard on the way to the top. 'I realised that if my happiness was contingent on my finding work as an actor, I was not going to be happy most of the time,' she writes in her autobiography, *Wake Up, I'm Fat*.[4] 'Every successful actor will tell you about the ten years when she couldn't even get arrested. Acting forces you to ask yourself "Can my constitution take a decade of constant rejection?"'

And rejection that was to be all the more lacerating because it was handed out on the grounds of Manheim's size, not her talent. Like many fat women, her parents were not able to validate her worth without conveying that she would be better if she lost weight. Her father even suggested she should smoke to help her lose it. 'All parents want their adult children to experience love, respect and lucrative employment, all of which my folks thought would be beyond my grasp if I didn't lose weight. I understand their concern. In fact, sadly, in many cases they are right. The world isn't lining up to love, respect and employ fat people.'

Manheim did lose weight, in a daze of drugs and promiscuity. Then clarity and reality intervened; she stopped the drugs and the gratuitous sex and regained the weight. What she also gained, for the first time, was a sense of identity: the foundation stone of the strong, powerful woman she is now.

> It finally occurred to me that when I'd lost the weight, I had lost myself. That conforming to a standard that was not developed with me in mind would be more counterproductive than good. I started to own my body, and I felt stronger and healthier than ever... There is nothing worse than being fat and hating yourself. I know. I lived there. But there is nothing more liberating than being fat and accepting yourself. It is the purest form of self-acceptance, loving yourself in a society that loathes you.'

It is clear from Manheim's story that she had a long struggle to reach an identity that allowed her to exploit her talent and her personality to the full. When you see her today, her confidence, her sense of mastery are very plainly authentic. She is at home in her body and in herself.

There are many strands to our identity; many faces that we present to the world. Some of us possess a greater number of masks than others; others, like Manheim, belong in the What You See is What You Get category.

My friend Pamela is like that. She is open, approachable and immediately friendly. She expects people to like her and they invariably do. When I wrote my first book on size prejudice[5] she was amazed. Not only did she feel she had not experienced prejudice herself, she claimed to be unaware that it existed at all!

I am 5′ 3″ and about 15 stone 11 lbs. Only in the last few years have I felt any embarrassment at my bulk as it seems to bulge now in the most unwelcome places – at least that is what the mirrors tell me. I was not always like this. I used to play lacrosse, hockey, cricket and netball at county level and much of my spare time was spent rushing around on my bike. Obviously, I believed I was good at sport and anyone who was sporty was popular. It never occurred to me that I might not be popular and, being extrovert, I never stopped to analyse my appearance or the impact I made when I walked into a room. I always tried to dress well and would never go outside without make-up – a habit I continue to this day. Even though I had gained a lot of weight over the years I did not think of myself as overweight and it has only been recently that I have dared to acknowledge that my weight is the same as that of those I consider to be obese. On the whole I do not like the appearance of the grossly overweight, especially if they do not dress well or they disdain make-up. I may be arrogant and I certainly am self-confident, which makes it difficult to face up to my size as being socially unacceptable. Do I think I have other loveable assets? Certainly. Am I insensitive to other people's impressions or opinions of me? Probably.

Pamela's sense of identity came first from possessing an ability – proficiency at sport – which not only made her feel accepted but also precluded the usual negative stereotypes being applied to her. When someone spends much of their time chasing a ball on a pitch it is impossible to accuse them of not getting up off their fat backside. They can hardly be called lazy. And it's clear that they are not lacking in self-discipline. Sporty people are generally seen as Good Eggs with Backbone, which may be a somewhat quirky mixed metaphor but it fits the bill!

So Pamela cruised through life, blissfully ignorant that she was a social misfit. She created a self-fulfilling prophecy: her high self-esteem and self belief was reflected in others' opinions and treatments of her. Nobody, it seemed, questioned her weight, least of all herself. Even when she gave up playing sport in her fifties and put on a large amount of weight, the consequences were to her physical not her emotional health. Her sense of her place in the world remained intact.

Yet it is obvious from Pamela's account that she is no anarchist. She feels she has to conform socially; it is just that her perception of what it means to conform has a different meaning. Make-up and a hairdresser-created coiffure are an essential part of her presentation to the world; without them she would certainly feel insecure and probably unacceptable. In fact, she has fairly rigid rules about personal appearance and admits that this is part of her identity: to be smart.

It is interesting that, although she acknowledges her large size – even admitting that she is the same as those she considers 'to be obese' – it is clear that she sees other fat women as somehow not like her. She says she does not like the appearance of the grossly overweight, especially if they are not smart and made-up (like her).

Though, like all of us, Pamela derives her sense of her identity from myriad different aspects of her self, her weight does not form part of it and in that she is unusual. She puts it down to not having been a fat child but I have not found that to be a reliable indicator of how people feel about their size. Indeed, I was a thin child until I was 11. I know that psychological theory would have it that your sense of self is laid down early, perhaps as early as five, but where size is concerned this does not seem to follow. Sometimes it can be exactly the reverse of what is expected: the thin child, the thin teenager perhaps, having established a sense of self embodied in that particular size and shape, then loses her sense of identity by becoming fat in adulthood. With that can go self-imposed shame and blame.

Fat – But Not Happy

This happened to Hilary:

> I was a really skinny child and I never gave my body a thought. When I was about 10, I started dancing seriously. I wanted to make a career of it. I remember the feeling of being able to make my body do what I wanted it to, to bend and twist and leap. I loved all that movement. As far as I remember I ate what I liked, just like any kid. In my teens I was dancing a lot, going out with boys, enjoying buying clothes, all the usual things.
>
> I got married in my twenties and had 4 children in 10 years. The weight piled on during my pregnancies but I was so busy with so many little ones that I didn't really notice it or do anything serious about it. When I was around 40 I hit a real crisis. My eldest daughter was 15 and we would go clothes shopping together. I realised that it had been a long time since I'd worn decent clothes and now I was so fat I didn't dare buy anything. Where had I gone? What had happened to *me*? I didn't know this fat person looking at me from changing-room mirrors. I hated her. I despised her. It had been a long time since I'd danced (I never did make a career of it but I had loved it until the babies came along). Now I realised that I couldn't dance even if I wanted to. My body seemed to roll, not move properly. It sickened me. I feel as though I've been two people. 'Normal' Hilary, who danced and laughed and lived life fully. She died, and along came fat Hilary who can't get it together. She stepped into normal Hilary's dead shoes like a kind of walk-in.
>
> I'm 50 now and still fat. I've dieted, of course – who hasn't? And put the weight back on – who hasn't done that, too? I rarely go out because I'm so ashamed of this foreign body. That's what it is. A foreign body is something that shouldn't be there, isn't it? Like a cockroach in the marmalade.

Hilary can acknowledge that she is a good mother, that she has skills and abilities and qualities that give her some sense of worth. But she has partly retired from the world because her late onset fat self is an unwelcome stranger to her. She doesn't know who she is because she grew up and lived part of her adult life as 'normal' Hilary. Unless she can reconcile 'normal' and 'fat' Hilary – or lose weight – she will continue to live with what she clearly sees as a split personality and this can only be destructive.

Annette deals with her size in a different way. As a young woman she was slim, successful and heading for the top. Then she was struck down by incapacitating agoraphobia, which necessitated abandoning her career and her jet-setting lifestyle. Addicted to the tranquillisers prescribed for her illness, she spent many years confined to the house – and she grew large. When she emerged from a 14-year fight with benzodiazepine addiction she felt she had missed out on everything: in particular the chance to marry and have a family. Now in her forties, this causes her a lot of pain.

It seemed that Annette lost all the markers of her identity: her job, her lifestyle, her confidence and her goals. But she has built a new career as a writer and PR consultant; she stays cheerful and positive and, most importantly, she believes in the benevolence of the future. Though motherhood will not be part of her defining identity as she always believed it would, she turns to other aspects of herself and builds on them. She will not let her size be a negative factor in her internal picture of who she is:

Butcher, baker, Monday's child. Er… Who am I? Philosophers and psychologists have already worked long and hard on this knotty question so I will leave the deeper side to more learned colleagues.

I am Annette. Right now I am overweight. I have had leaner times but for various reasons this isn't one of them. Now if we were talking about height I couldn't say, 'Actually this is a short time but with determination I have every confidence in soon gaining a few inches.' I am five feet tall and sadly, at age 44, I think my upward growing spurt is over.

This Annette is always going to be five feet tall and there is only one way forward and to a great extent it applies to life in general: we have to make the most of it and deal with the cards, not bemoan what we were dealt. For me this means making the best of what I have. I like my straight nose, warm eyes and thick hair. I care for my skin with lotions and potions, paint my toenails, use the best French perfume, buy flowers every week and cook for friends with love.

I think part of my identity now is being plump and I can't imagine what it would be like not to have a cleavage or a bonny face. That this offends people is ridiculous. After having highlights put in my hair, I whizzed into the local deli for some cream (kedgeree for a supper party). 'You'll be wanting the low fat,' said the shopkeeper. There was another lady, a thin one, in the store who could have understudied for Worzel Gummidge. Did anyone spray air freshener, refer to the state of her hair, suggest she had breast implants or a nose job? No, she just got served her chocolate and cheeses.

So many assumptions are made about being overweight. It isn't a licence to slob out and I stay healthy by walking. It isn't a reason to take a rain check on the beauty products or not to buy clothes. But whatever our size, physical pluses or minuses, I think we all have a responsibility to be our personal best and I guess what I present to the world is that I am trying. Things are far from perfect but what percentage of the population would pass muster as a supermodel?

Indeed. And when I consider the issues explored in Chapter One – the discontent that the size-12 woman feels about her 'fat' body; the secret longing to be not just thin but *too* thin experienced by the most politically aware, mature and intelligent women; the sense of dismay that runs through female society because the right degree of thinness just seems too unattainable – then I feel a huge surge of pride and admiration for women like Annette, who are able to love their unsociable bodies just as they are and to treat them well.

Diana Pollard, founder of SIZE, is honest, realistic and also totally self-accepting, but she admits to what many size-acceptance activists would deny: a desire to be less fat. This is because she is an eminently practical woman and is not afraid to say what many of us feel: that life would be easier, physically and socially, if she were not as large as she is.

I have never wanted to be thin but I have wanted to be slimmer than I am. I'd rather not be this large. Would I take a magic pill?

If I could take a harmless magic pill to make me thin I would but I wouldn't want to stay thin so I'd then work at trying to get a bit bigger. I'd eat healthily until I got myself to a comfortable size. If there was a safe way of losing weight without drugs or surgery or starvation, of course I'd take it. I'd rather be several sizes smaller than I am. I'm someone who eats a healthy diet. I exercise within my limitations.

I've always been more self-conscious about my crooked, lopsided body and my limp. I'd love to have a matching pair of legs. Before I was fat I was easily identifiable as having a disability. But now people see my fatness first. As a fat person I'm not condescended to; I'm insulted, I am abused, ignored, judged, but people are not benevolent towards me the way they used to be.

I'm a great one for self-nurturing. I love nice clothes. I love sensual fabrics. I spend a small fortune on indulgences for the bath. I love being massaged and I look after my skin. In 1996, I had a set of nude drawings done of me by Sarah Alec and that was a nice thing to do. Unless I had felt comfortable with her I wouldn't have wanted her to draw me. I'm proud of those drawings.

I'm a friend to my body. My body is troublesome. I've never had a healthy body – and I spent a large part of my life as a slim child. In adulthood I started to gain weight. I've spent a lot of my life coaxing my body to do things. I've got bigger over the years and there have been times when I've felt desperately betrayed by my body. 'How could you do this to me when I've put such good food into you and I've tried to do so many things to help you and you respond by abusing my trust and my good nature.' But I go on being a friend to it. Considering I came into the world in such an unhealthy state I suppose that's where the pride comes in. Sometimes I find it awesome that I've managed to achieve so much in this body. I feel it's covered in battlescars but still somehow roadworthy. If I could have exactly what I want in a perfect world I'd be smaller but it' s not a perfect world. I never rule out the possibility of my body changing for the better. I'm always working towards improving my health but I do love myself. Sometimes I talk to my body as if it's a disobedient child: 'However naughty you are I'll go on loving you but sometimes you make it very hard for me to love you.

I feel a sense of enormous joy and homecoming when I encounter the unusual fat woman who truly loves herself, who is so *bien dans sa peau* that her feeling of wholeness, of being fully her *self* communicates itself so strongly that you can begin to feel it, too. The American novelist Susan Stinson is like that. She is someone I study with envy for she is such a rarity.

This is what she says about being fat:

I love my body. I love it with the force of a basic impulse towards self-preservation, with an animal appreciation for what my bones, joints, tendons, muscles, organs, veins, skin and fat can do. There are neglected symphonies of meaning in all my belly does for supporting and sustaining breath, for yielding pleasure in sex, and for facilitating the transformation of food into the energy needed for every human action. Mouth, tongue, eyes, wrists, fingertips: every element of the body could be a poem and a treatise. Fat has its place among them.

I love my body as a political act, a daily affirmation of the idea that the world can change to include things as difficult to envision as more equitable distribution of power and resources, and appreciation for a wide range of bodies, including mine. Each time I move with pleasure, dress myself comfortably, or offer my physical self a moment of praise, it is an act of homage to people all over the world who have faced difficult circumstances and taken steps to change them. My small, personal acts of resistance are not in themselves full expressions of my support for others whose bodies and lives are treated with disrespect, but they help keep me awake to how difficult and how important those struggles are.

I love my body as a spiritual discipline, a way of knowing myself and my surroundings. I try to experience my physical sensations as directly as I can, and to notice when distractions are getting in the way. Fear of death is, I find, a large distraction. So is a longing to be accepted by a culture which rejects me as an unworthy participant because I am a fat woman. It's very difficult for me to accept changes in my body, to face pain, illness, imperfection. There is a temptation to believe that these things are my fate because I am a fat woman, but it appears to me that they are part of the human condition.

It's difficult to resist the fat hatred that the culture directs at me in terms of economic and social discrimination, limited accessibility and biased health care. It's hard to be joyful, tender and healthy under the stress of all that. The strength of other fat people who resist these pressures sustains me. The struggle to love my body is worth the risk and effort it takes. And I do. I love my lush, soft, fat body as it swells every space I enter with its undeniable, vibrant presence.

In 1996, Susan came to stay with me when she came to this country to promote her beautiful novel, *Martha Moody*.[6] The heroine of her book is like Susan herself and I recommend it for its beauty, its fine writing and its joyful portrayal of a fat woman. This is how I reviewed *Martha Moody*:

This is a story about love and friendship and loss, about reconciliation, understanding and about finally coming home. In the two central characters, Martha and Amanda, we see the strength and tenacity of feisty women pitted against the rough judgment of men and of a small nineteenth-century community whose upright inhabitants are committed to the upholding of temperance and fundamental Christianity.

Martha Moody is magnificent. She is unashamedly fat and she is beautiful, dignified and desirable. She will take her place in modern literature as a truly marvellous role model for large women. I loved the image of her in church 'filling half the pew with her flesh and God's grace'. Never before have I encountered the large body depicted with such beauty. What woman would not want to be 'soft in mounds and extravagant in flesh?' With this novel, Susan Stinson has glorified the large female body, and without overstatement she conveys that fatness and sexuality are joyfully and inextricably bound up together and that abundance of female flesh is a celebration and a delight.

I noticed that Susan held herself differently from most fat women. She stood tall, instead of hunching, or folding in on herself. Her movements were fluid, sinuous, balletic. I was mesmerised by the poetic rhythms of her grace, the kind of natural freedoms we associate with large Afro-Caribbean women but not with those from our own western culture. This was beauty in action and it was hard to imagine Susan as thinner: just trying to do so brought to mind visions of angularity and gaucheness.

I became conscious of the way my posture had developed over the years into a defensive, protective shield, as though if I hid my body no one would notice that I was fat. I could not seem to relax, to let my arms move in harmony with my body. I was not at home in my own skin.

There is no doubt that our identity, our vision of who we are, is inseparably bound up with our size and I am fascinated by those women whose largeness is an essential part of that identity. Sheila Kitzinger, the childbirth educator, is another such woman. Her role as helpmeet to women in labour, women in prison, women seeking asylum, is one that is concomitant with her generous, enfolding earth motherliness. But it also confers a sense of authority: 'I could not sweep onto a platform to give a lecture if I were not this size,' she says. 'I would not have the presence. And I would not feel right wearing my capes!'

Sheila's capes are silk, handpainted by her with birth symbols, explicit images of vulvas and vaginas, outrageous but appropriate, eccentric but beautiful. Sheila's life and her work celebrate fecundity, ampleness, growth, fruition. A thin Sheila Kitzinger would not have the impact she does. As for health: this woman has so much energy that she leaves you gasping and trailing in her wake! She has asthma but it does not slow her. When she turned seventy I asked her if she was going to take life a bit easier. 'Yes,' she said. 'I am now getting up at six instead of five.'

Jill Welbourne is someone else whose sense of self, of strength and authority is vested in her size.

Doctors say I should lose at least two stone. I'm fifteen stone and 5′ 9″. I can't afford to lose two stone; I need my weight. I need every ounce of it to throw around! I had a nightmare the other night and in the nightmare I was thinner and I couldn't get people to listen to me and I woke up actually saying 'I can't afford to lose weight. I need my power.' There are words like presence and gravitas and authority which go with weight. It is a comfort to know that if I'm dealing with someone who is dotty I can push her into a chair and say sit down, and have enough weight to get her to sit down without being pushed over by her when she's barging around. I'm very much considered overweight, in the slightly obese category. Fifteen stone is an Edwardian weight that gives me a décolletage without salt cellars. If I'm normal weight, I'm scrawny and have ribs showing and look all hunched and out of proportion. At this weight I am in proportion. I am much more comfortable and life is socially much easier, being all of a piece.

These women are wonderful role models. But we cannot all feel the same, however passionately we believe in size-acceptance issues. Some of us do not have such a well-developed sense of self; why this should be is academic and probably irrelevant to this part of the debate.

Belinda Charlton, who was once very fat and who lost 12 stone to run the London Marathon, feels just the opposite to Jill and Sheila:

I followed a vicious circle of dieting, failing and then comfort eating until I became gross [22 stone] and then very ill. In the process I discovered that 'big' is invisible. When you grow as big as I did people make you feel you do not exist. I was ignored, as people ignore waiters. Eyes slid past me to focus on someone else. I was edited out of mind, made to feel part of the wallpaper. In response I tried to make myself unobtrusive, to withdraw into the sanctuary of anonymity.

So Belinda, in her own mind, ceased to exist. (The rest of her story is told in Chapter Seven.) This is a frightening aspect of fat identity: so powerful are the messages that we should *not* exist that many of us try to fade out of mainstream life.

However, Lee Kennedy feels all *too* visible – in the wrong way, to the wrong people – and it is invisibility that she seeks:

I can't blame my obesity for my chronic unhappiness. If I could be free of it, though, I do feel I would suffer less from the very real abuse I have had to endure over the years through not looking passable – not having to brace myself for the stares, remarks, loud harassment by youths, etc, that the obese have to put up with, every time I go outdoors. It would be so sweet not to be *noticed* in that way. I have often *seriously considered* buying a chador to wear on those days when I find going out almost too much to contemplate. I may actually do it, some day – voluntarily put myself in purdah just for the bliss of not being hassled about my appearance.

One of the most difficult things for fat women to contend with can be large breasts. They get in the way. Wearing a bra is uncomfortable; not wearing a bra can be *extremely* uncomfortable. Many of us wear the wrong size; we are far too embarrassed to get measured properly.

We cannot choose to hide our breasts under loose clothes because if they are very big, nothing will conceal them. More often than not they give out messages we would rather they didn't. Few large women opt for breast reduction because of the fear of medical prejudice and the risk of an operation.

Lee Kennedy did, though. It did nothing for her already low self-esteem that, as a young woman, the wrong sort of men were attracted to her.

That's when The Tits became an issue. Dear old mum had often expressed the hope that I wouldn't get 'too big in the bust' as both my nans had been. Of course I sprouted a gigantic pair, as if cursed by the Tit Fairy, and spent the next four decades grimly seeking ways to disguise them. One of the grossest things about them was that they seemed to appeal to some 'lower-class' oafish males, while the arty swots I lusted for, and could actually communicate with on most levels, only wanted slender, elegant girls with the fronts of their bright little shift dresses all gorgeously flat. I developed an increasingly warped attitude as I went though many one-night stands with men I found extremely unappealing, knowing that *they* were only with *me* because they couldn't do better for themselves. The only thing my partners usually had in common, apart from being unattractive, was their perverse enthusiasm for my monstrous Irish tits...

Lee could not afford to have the operation privately and had to wait until she was in her fifties to have an NHS reduction. With an understanding GP she had the surgery with no size-related problems, though she could not persuade the surgeon to give her her 'dream since adolescence' – to make her totally flat-chested. In spite of the fact that her reduced breasts were severely asymmetrical, requiring yet more surgery, Lee is 'euphoric'.

Sometimes the stress of living in a fat-hating society is so consuming that even in death many fat people fear that they will not be equal or acceptable. They have visions of a giant-width coffin carried by extra ranks of bearers; they imagine the disapproving cluckings from the assembled mourners as the doughty coffin-shoulderers bow under the load. If you are above a certain weight you cannot opt for the environmentally friendly cardboard coffin – it may give way.

There is an unbearably poignant scene in the film *What's Eating Gilbert Grape?* when the eponymous protagonist's very large mother dies. This woman is depicted as someone so terrifyingly large that her very size endangers the house's foundations. When she dies in her bed upstairs, the family is informed that her body will have to be removed by a crane. Gilbert, unable to cope with such humiliation, burns down the house with their mother's body inside.

This film, with its portrayal of a fat woman as a dysfunctional yet pathetic object, touches the deepest parts of our fears: that even in death we may not be accorded the dignity given to the favoured thin.

Lee Kennedy expresses this fear in graphic terms:

I also have a morbid terror of *dying* fat – stuff I've read over the years about the gruesome properties of obese corpses haunts me – it would be so humiliating to explode, be preserved in my own fat, etc, etc (as if even thin corpses were superior, or that I was actually going to be there to be embarrassed by my coarse style of decomposition!).

Fatness and Affluence

Only a very tiny percentage of the world has adequate food: a shocking fact that most of us choose not to think about for much of the time because of the distress and guilt it can induce. In addition, it is far from comfortable to confront the issues of fatness and capitalism. We know about the African fattening houses; we know that once fatness was prized in many cultures because it was a marker of wealth, of ability to provide – of having 'made it' in a society where most people did not.

Those criteria have been somewhat turned on their head: it is now the poorest people (in western society) who are fat because junk food is cheaper than fresh food. Nevertheless, there is an association between fatness, greed, excess and over-abundance that makes us squirm. It is almost impossible to be a fat person and not to hear a voice whispering in your ear 'You have eaten too much'.

Addie Estey, a Canadian film maker who is fat herself, finds it hard to come to terms with these juxtapositions. Here she refers to a newspaper article that made her uneasy:

It was about meat addicts – a woman whose columns I actually quite like usually (she quotes Huxley without explaining who he is, and I appreciate that sort of vote of confidence) had had some sort of traumatic event at a steak house, watching enormously fat people plow through huge steaks soaked in butter. It was essentially her way of saying she was done eating red meat, and that she thought North Americans in particular were killing themselves with their 'addiction' to same.

I understand the columnist's problem with the meat, but she alluded to that scene in Monty Python's *The Meaning of Life* when the enormous man eats and vomits all over the restaurant – you know it? As graphic a metaphor for capitalism as you're likely to ever see – and one that haunts me.

Society tells us it's our fault we're fat – if we were just stronger, we'd thin up. It also tells us we deserve pleasure, and when we deserve pleasure, it can take the form of junk food. And in our sadness at hearing the first message, we embrace the second – and eat garbage, and get fatter. Not all of us – some of us would be stout no matter what we did – but particularly in North America, where bad food is plentiful and cheap, we end up feeding the corporate machines that profit by feeding us crap.

But what do we do about the gluttons? You know who I mean, I've got one in my family – a huge waddling child of a man with an irritating chuckle, who crams all manner of horrific things into his mouth because he can: because he's got the money, because as a white male North American he's pretty much won the evolutionary food race, and now he can just sate himself on empty food. He's not sad, he's greedy. He's not compulsive, he's self-indulgent. He's every fat activist's nightmare I imagine – the equivalent of the black junkie pimp for the civil rights movement.

His size *is* a product of lack of moral fibre! And there is a moral problem with a society that is so affluent, and so blind to the hunger and poverty of the rest of the world, that it eats itself into inertia, and then dumps the waste of its gorging in countries starving for a fraction of the food squandered here.

I'm fat – and I'm repelled by that image. I don't think my fatness is a product of excess now, but certainly as a North American it may have its roots there. How do I learn to think of my body as being part of a spectrum of perfectly normal body types, when I'm revolted by the gluttony of my culture?

I am wrestling with this knot all the time. Is 'celebrate' the right word to use around fatness? Should it be more 'understand' – the way we understand alcoholics and drug addicts, as long as they're trying to keep straight? Are there different kinds of fatness? The 'can't be helped – genetic – if you're mean to me you're a bigot' fatness, and then other, less worthy of celebration kinds?

In tackling head-on the issue of fatness and greed, Addie Estey presents an uncomfortable but necessary aspect of the debate. When you look at this aspect, the trivial matter of what is fashionable or aesthetically prescribed loses any significance. Whatever the reason for our fatness, the truth is that we are going to be judged by most people by the harshest of standards and the assumption of our greed will be implicit in that judgment, even though it is sometimes unconscious.

If fat people are not to be seen as greedy, should they allow themselves to be seen as disabled? Feelings run high on this issue within the size-acceptance movement. There is no doubt that above a certain weight some fat people *are* disabled, just as some fat people are greedy. As a group in society we are not claiming to be perfectly adjusted, physically fit, morally sound human beings.

So should there be virtue in fatness acquired through certain identifiable causes? Personally, I have always felt that there should not be exceptions. A size-acceptance magazine I once worked for wanted me to write a piece on non-self-induced fat – but I felt very strongly that this would not sit well with the ethos of the magazine. If you say that some people are large because of certain diseases or (prescription) drugs – therefore it is not their fault – what is that saying about everyone else? To me this is rather like sympathising only with the 'innocent' victims of AIDS.

I agree with Addie Estey that 'celebrate' is a difficult word to use around fatness. But then I don't agree with celebrating thinness either. What I would like is for both thinness and fatness to be irrelevant, but as long as these states are so densely saturated with moral connotations, this will not happen.

The Fat Person's Place in Society

The question of identity has much to do with validation from the society in which we live. We soon learn what is good and what is bad, which is why a strong, anarchic tendency is such a must for a fat person. But we also need to see positive aspects of our selves reflected back to us.

Where *do* we see positive images of fat people reflected back? Not in places of power and influence on the whole. Ann Widdecombe gets away with it – though many see her as a caricature, an object of derision. Jackie Ballard, MP for Taunton and one-time Liberal Democrat leadership contender, bowed to the pressure, lost weight and was the happier for it. Nigel Lawson became more famous for his vast weight loss than he ever did as a politician.

And these images are not to be found (with the exceptions detailed in Chapter One, of course) in the media, in fashion and in most of the professions. When I worked for BBC Radio 4 as a presenter and producer I was aware that promotion was passing me by. I did not understand; I knew I was good at what I did because I'd had enough feedback for me not to be in any doubt. But I was told that I was being held back because of my weight. One well-known presenter had complained about me going on location. What I was told was that I didn't 'present a good image of the BBC'. I was told I had to lose weight if I wanted to get anywhere.

Talk about identity crisis. Where was 'I' in all this? What about the quality of my work and the fact that I had the ability to make people relaxed, thus getting good interviews from them? Was that presenting 'a bad image'? This was *radio*, for God's sake! In those days I had no concept of the politics of size acceptance though the experience sowed the seeds from which my later work grew. But I left the BBC, my spirit crushed.

Employers are afraid that the negative qualities associated with fatness – greed, idleness, sloppiness, lack of discipline, of purpose and self-respect – will by association be attributed to the company that employs fat people. There is absolutely no proof that any of these stereotypes are justified but it makes no difference. When people do see a fat glutton (as opposed to a thin glutton; they certainly exist but pass unnoticed) the stereotype springs into being. One sighting is enough to condemn everyone else by association.

If a fat person does make it, his/her size will always be commented on – not just once but constantly. Even if that person is praised, even if s/he is described as smart, good-looking, clever, an achiever, there is a subtext: *in spite of being fat*. It is never allowed to go without comment. It is never allowed to be irrelevant.

Though this is entirely the fault of the society we live in, not the fat person, it does make it harder to form a solid sense of identity. When the person you are feels obliterated by an attack on something that should have nothing to do with who you are, when the society you live in does not represent you, even while it delights in telling you that you make up a large and growing percentage of the population, it does, almost inevitably, influence the way you feel about yourself. If, on top of this, your peers, your family or your friends confirm these messages by suggesting, albeit ever so nicely, that it would be better – *you* would be better – if you lost weight, it is hard to know where to turn for support. Even many fat people are prejudiced.

The thing about being overweight is that it is never out of your mind. You don't adapt to it, you don't forget about it or become accustomed to it like wearing glasses or dentures. You are conscious of your body every day in every way. You are conscious of it physically because the human skeleton was not designed to carry so much flesh and our working, domestic and social environments are not designed to contain it. Unless you are superbly fit, you are aware that you cannot run for the bus or climb five flights of stairs like those of normal weight.

When, in addition to value judgments, you see no place for you either – when seating is too meagre; when it's hard to get decent, large-sized clothes in spite of the fact that size 16 is the *average* size for a woman in Britain; when going for a hospital check-up is an ordeal because their ridiculous gowns won't meet round you – you could be forgiven for wondering whether you actually *exist*.

It is unlikely that in the foreseeable future there will be legislation to protect the rights of the overweight. We do not have a Commission for Size Equality, nor will we. At the moment the law-makers are as prejudiced as everyone else, therefore few see it as a valid civil or human rights issue.

Size and Self-worth

I recognise that I am not a Susan Stinson or a Sheila Kitzinger, much as I would like to be. I find it impossible to feel good about myself when I am a very high weight. I do not want to leave this chapter without giving a voice to someone who feels very differently from me. The following is a dialogue between myself and Jill Welbourne, which gives our two different views of fat identity:

Shelley: What about the person who weighs 20 stone and cannot accept herself at that weight?

Jill: Someone who cannot accept her weight is divided from herself. The genes are settled – a given. Eighty per cent of eventual height and weight is determined by genes. Attempts to reshape oneself through diet and exercise are only trimming. There is nothing you can do about it. To hate what is the scaffolding of your body, the house of your soul, the place where you live, your locating signal in the world, is idiotic.

Shelley: How can you be at home in your body if you are very fat and vulnerable to the censure of others?

Jill: Can you take charge of the thoughts in other people's heads? No. So why exhaust yourself trying to control other people's thoughts? Say this over and over again as a mantra: 'I give you permission to have any opinion at all because I let you. Because I am permitting you to have this freedom, I have more control. It is my decision, my choice that you may think what you like.' It's hard to apply but if you keep on saying it you actually become far less worried about what other people think. Then you have greater freedom, you have the chance of finding out what *you* want.

Shelley: It's very hard to convince people that they have the right to be themselves.

Jill: What choices do they feel they've got? You have to live with yourself twenty-four hours a day, seven days a week. You cannot get away from yourself so there is no point in saying things to yourself that increase your misery. You have to learn to be an encouraging, supportive, optimistic friend to yourself. If you're sitting there saying 'I'm a hideous size and I hate it' you're not being a friend to yourself. So say 'I wish I weren't this size but I don't think there's anything I can do to change it and what can't be cured instantly must be endured for today, so I'll make myself comfortable today' you are. Being comfortable in every sense is important for psychological well-being and that includes physical comfort too – like having the right posture, like wearing a well-fitting, supporting bra and clothes that you like.

This is good psychological common sense. Like Lee Kennedy, I envy those like Jill who can give the finger to the abusers. But there is no point in trying to adopt a spurious confidence: it doesn't work. I tried it for years, letting people think I was quite happy with my size, that I knew who I was without having to change myself for the benefit of others. This is not the place for an analysis of what bestows confidence and how deep its roots are. I only know that people like me and Lee Kennedy (and actually, most women if truth be told) are the majority and those like Jill – who has the most supreme self-belief of anyone I've ever met, man or woman – are the lucky minority.

I know my worth does not depend on my weight but many people are not able to think of themselves in this way, perhaps because they do not have the loving, accepting, non-judgmental support system that I do. It's tough living in a society that hates you and no amount of belief in the wrongness of prejudice changes that fact. Early size-acceptance pioneers used to make the comparison with race, saying that 'you wouldn't expect a black person to bleach their skin – until it became apparent that this was *exactly* what some black people were doing. The single most difficult thing about establishing a positive sense of identity as a fat person is that unlike other oppressed groups we are seen to possess the power to change, whether that is real or illusory.

Size Acceptance and Weight Loss Are Not Mutually Exclusive

I firmly believe that changing your body size is not the answer to prejudice. But I have spoken to and received letters from women far too unhappy to have acceptance urged upon them. Since my first enthusiastic, campaigning book was published,[7] I have encountered pain that cannot be ameliorated by politics. Some women just cannot bear their fat bodies and this *must* be respected by fat-hating bigots and fat activists alike.

So weight loss must be an option for some women. This is what Jill Welbourne says about the need to be thinner:

It is only when you accept you can't change that you are free to change. Only when you think it isn't going to happen, you're going to be this size – and then one day you think I'm not sure I'm going to be this size – I'll see. But you have to get to that point of acceptance before you can lose weight successfully. It's only when you are prepared to be big that you can actually start to be slimmer.

For my own part, I'm claiming a halfway victory, an ambivalence. My identity is tied up with being a caregiver. My role as a mother is the most important one in my life; it is where I feel the most comfortable and fulfilled. As a mother – to my children obviously, but also to any stray lame dogs – I am an earth mother. Like Jill, I would say I need my weight. I don't think earth mothers can be thin, but I desperately wanted to be less fat. I weighed over 19 stone and I didn't feel like me. I knew that I wouldn't feel like me at 9 stone either, but that 12^1/$_2$ would be nice. Very overweight for my height, 12^1/$_2$ stone.

So, against all my previous principles, I dieted and lost six and a half stone. And here I have to disagree with Jill. It was only when I could bear it no longer that I was able to believe that I could do something about it. One of my codes for living is that 'there is a solution to everything'. My solution was to think that if 95 people out of 100 regain the weight they lose, why should I not be one of the five who don't?

Chapter Four
Why Do We Get Fat?

It's in the Genes

Fatness is considered to be a multifactorial condition – an ongoing nature versus nurture debate – but one clear fact has emerged in the last few years. Fatness is genetic. If you have become fat, environmental factors will certainly have played a part, but you would not have done so without a strong genetic predisposition.

Obesity does tend to run in families. Where both parents are fat, their children have a 70 per cent chance of becoming fat, compared to the children of non-fat parents who have a less than 20 per cent chance. Some have attempted to explain this by pointing out that children and parents are likely to share the same lifestyle patterns: in this case too much of the wrong food and not enough exercise. But observation of adopted children shows that they are more likely to conform to their natural parents' weights than those of the family they are brought up in. The most compelling examples of this are to be found in identical twins reared separately.

The obesity, or *ob* gene was first described in 1994 and was located in genetically obese mice. The gene was found to control the production of leptin, which regulates appetite and satiety. When the mice were given injections of leptin they stopped overeating, increased their energy expenditure and lost weight. It is not that simple for us. Human obesity is likely to involve more than one gene and scientists have yet to isolate them, though it is believed that a preference for a sedentary lifestyle or for high-fat foods is also genetically determined.[1]

It seems that overweight humans, like the fat mice, don't know when they have eaten sufficient; they don't recognise satiety. This becomes a chicken and egg situation: you get fat because your calorie intake is too great; your calorie intake is too great because you don't have the mechanism to regulate it: you diet, which then throws a spanner in the works because of the famine response galvanised into action through dieting. Once the famine response

is switched on you have little chance of recognising physical
satiety until you are overfull.

Now, you cannot blame a mouse for becoming fat. You cannot
accuse a mouse of greed, sloth, lack of will power or lack of self-
discipline. The leptin research is exciting, not least because it
should absolve those who are fat. Even if they are fat through what
is perceived, by our social rulebook, as greed, that excess should
not be seen as morally reprehensible if they have a faulty satiety
mechanism.

Just as an aside, one researcher remarked to me that the odd
thing was that the obese mice were far more attractive and
appealing than their 'normal' thin counterparts. They were
cuddly and friendly, he said, they were nicer looking and more
likeable.

It is true, in a very literal sense, that people who gain very large
amounts of weight do so by 'overeating', but this word needs
careful analysis. In its literal sense, it means that some people take
in too many calories for their own particular, individual, metabolic
energy requirements. Those requirements may be very low and
may not match appetite or normal patterns of eating. I am happy
to say that at least one obesity expert does not allow the word
'overeating' to be used in connection with his patients. Dr Julian
Barth, who runs an obesity clinic at the Leeds General Infirmary,
feels that the word is too judgmental. The moral connotations of
it are entirely pejorative.[2]

I know I have these genes. I have always been fascinated by
watching people of 'normal' weight eating. They start a meal then
they start to slow down. Then, usually while chatting, not even
consciously noticing what they are doing, they put their knife and
fork together. There is still food on their plate but they have
finished. They have had enough and they don't have a starved,
panicky voice in their head saying, 'You can't leave that, there
might not be any more where that came from.' They don't even
think about it. If their satiety mechanism has kicked in they can
see no point in going on eating.

My theory is that a genetic predisposition by itself would
probably not make people *very* fat, though it is difficult to give
definitive weights. I believe my own genes would have caused me
to be about 11 stone (at 5' 3") if other factors like repeated

dieting had not entered the equation. However much I try to dispute obesity research, where the emphasis seems to be on blaming the individual, it is an inescapable truth that the huge increase in obesity – both in degree and prevalence – over the last 50 years cannot be purely genetic. It is too short a period in evolutionary terms and the genepool has remained essentially constant in that time.[3]

So, given that the genetic predisposition must exist first, what else makes us fat?

The Influence of Culture and Society

It cannot be insignificant that the increase in the incidence of obesity coincides with the cultural insistence on a thin body and the corresponding growth in all forms of dieting. Fifty years ago it was unusual to see people of very high weights; fifty years ago the thin aesthetic had not become mandatory.

This is what I believe is one of the main causes of obesity today: repeated low-calorie dieting. There is an ongoing battle between many obesity researchers and those who have dieted because of the stubborn insistence on the part of many of the pundits that dieting does not cause subsequent weight gain. They back up their argument by asserting that cultures which experience cycles of plenty and famine do not have messed up metabolisms. But this is far too simplistic. In such circumstances, people cannot choose the type and quantity of food; their intake is dictated by availability. They do get fatter in times of plenty but the cycles are regular and there is never enough to get very fat. But tribal obesity is not unknown and the American Pima Indians illustrate what can happen when food shortage is followed by unlimited availability.

The Pima tribes split into two groups: one in Arizona, the other in Mexico. Genetically, they are identical. The Arizona Pimas hit a major crisis at the beginning of the twentieth century when white settlers diverted the course of the river on Pima territory. The land grew barren and the tribe suffered from poverty, malnutrition and starvation. There were many, many deaths and the Pimas desperately struggled to maintain their very existence. Then in 1984 the tribe was granted a casino concession. Money flowed, they became affluent, they took jobs in the business. And they joined mainstream American society, embracing the lifestyle – and the high-fat, fast-food diet.

The result of this was that this branch of the Pima tribe became the fattest population group in the United States. Their incidence of the diseases traditionally associated with obesity is staggering: 50 per cent of the adult Pima population is diabetic. The other splinter of the tribe remains in Mexico, living on subsistence farming. They are not fat.

This is not an isolated incidence of fatness following famine in the cultural rather than the elective sense. The anthropologist Margaret Mackenzie has noticed similar patterns when other cultures migrate to the West and adopt its lifestyle.[4]

But the Pimas give the most dramatic example of the effects of feast following famine. Surely this suggests that the same cause and effect will be found whatever the reason for the shortage?

Almost all diets are low calorie because their proponents are offering quick weight loss. Even the prescribed, medically acceptable reduction of 2 lbs per week is a fast weight loss and one that the body will not take kindly to. With rare exceptions, if you follow a diet below 1400–1500 calories a day you will not be getting enough to eat. Your body thinks it is in famine. But because of the ready availability of food in our society, your body will not allow you to be hungry and will simply override your will power. Every single diet that is too low in calories ends in a binge and more weight gain per calorie because of the famine effect. It would appear that dieting can indeed make you fat.

The Effects of a Modern Lifestyle

I have a book on nutrition and cookery published in the fifties which makes astonishing reading today, when obesity, anorexia, junk food and orthorexia (an obsession with eating correct foods) are all part of the chaotic jumble which constitutes modern eating.

A balanced diet, says this book, must contain Protective Foods (dairy foods, vegetables and fruit, fat fish – what we call oily fish); Body-building Foods (meat, milk, eggs, cheese, fish); and Foods for Calories (dripping, frying fats, suet, butter, margarine, bacon, cheese, cereals, cakes, biscuits, bread, pastry, pulses, dried fruits, jam, marmalade, golden syrup, treacle, potatoes).

We should eat five meals a day: breakfast, elevenses, lunch, tea and supper.

The author states that 'calories (ie the fuel value of foods) will usually look after themselves: so long as the eater is healthy and contented and leads a reasonable life, with plenty of fresh air and exercise. Normal appetite leads a person to eat enough and not too much or too little.'

Elevenses should consist of 'coffee dash' – whole milk with just a dash of coffee – and biscuits. There is a tempting photograph of 'A well-balanced tea, with egg and cress sandwiches, bread and butter and jam and cake.'

The book gives four weeks of suggested menus, divided into seasons. It is easy to forget, in this age of total availability, that not so very long ago people did have to depend on the natural rhythms of the year; there was no importing of strawberries in January. Even bananas were quite a luxury.

This is a menu for an autumn day:

Breakfast	Lunch	Tea	Supper
Cereal	Grilled Cutlets with	Egg and Shredded	Asparagus Soup
Fried Brains	Julienne Potatoes	Lettuce Sandwiches	Braised Calf'sTongue
Bread and	Cabbage	Walnut Cake	Spinach
Marmalade	Steamed Fig	Sponge Cake	Mashed Potatoes
or Honey	Pudding and Custard		Cornflour Pudding

My 87-year-old mother-in-law always produced meals to this pattern and she never got bigger than a size 10. My healthily brought up children used to beg to be taken there for tea, where they had Mr Kipling cakes, chocolate fingers and fruit cake with cherries in it. It was such a treat that for every birthday I made them a Granny Tea, a tradition which lasted until they flew the nest and no longer celebrated birthdays at home.

Granny, who had a weakness for cakes and who would eat chocolates in between times, never put on an ounce. But Granny also went for long, fast dog walks three times a day with my children running on little legs to keep up with her. She nipped around all day doing housework, gardening, washing and ironing and only sat down for prescribed short periods – no slobbing out in front of the telly. I now know, from studying the energy burned in that kind of activity, that she was using up hundreds of calories every day. She is not unusual: she is a product of her generation.

Before the sixties, people both consumed and burned many more calories than we do today. It may sound an over-simplification to say it's a lifestyle thing but it certainly plays a part.

The Toxic Food Environment

There is also no doubt that modern, western lifestyle has been one of the major causes of the current prevalence of very high weight. There is too much food to choose from and too much of it is junk. In America it is difficult to get anything to eat in a 'normal' size. Everything is supersized and there are more supersized people in America than anywhere else in the world.

We are surrounded by high-fat, high-calorie, high-sugar, over-processed and denatured food. Few people cook and eat using fresh ingredients. In short, according to Professor Kelly Brownell, director of the Yale Centre for Eating and Weight Disorders, we are living in a toxic food environment.[5] Much of this food is available cheaply from fast food outlets and it tastes pretty good to most people. It's not difficult to eat a lot of it, especially when everything seems to come with 'extras': extra cheese in your double cheeseburger, extra relish, extra fries.

Brownell describes a typical 'toxic food environment' near his office.

If I drive down that road for just ten minutes I pass about 30 different places where one could get highly processed, high-calorie, high-fat food. There are fast-food restaurants that are open 24 hours, ones that have drive-through facilities so that you don't even have to get out of your car to get a meal, places that offer 'all you can eat' buffets for an inclusive low price, service stations that have been remodelled with mini-markets inside, and all promoting high-fat food at low cost.[6]

There is no doubt at all that eating that kind of food will make people fat. But is toxic food environment a bit of dramatic overstatement? I don't think so. Especially when you discover the true nature of what you are eating.

In a book that makes horrifically compulsive reading, the truth about fast-food preparation is revealed.[7]

The food served in burger joints must be heavily processed in order to achieve uniformity. The natural flavour of the ingredients is removed and replaced with chemicals. For instance, barbecue flavours are created by charring sawdust, capturing the aroma chemicals in water and then bottling it. A Burger King strawberry milkshake contains more than 50 chemical flavours.

Fast-food processing is a sophisticated science. Not only is taste an issue, but mouthfeel is artificially created, too. A mechanical 'mouth' full of probes tests food for bounce, density, crunchiness, juiciness, spreadability and tackiness amongst other things

The McDonald's handbook for employees is called the Bible and runs to nearly 800 pages. It contains exact instructions about everything: the thickness of chips, how far apart burgers should be placed on a grill. Not conforming to these instructions can lead to loss of franchise. Ray Kroc, one of the marketing brains behind McDonald's, said: 'We cannot trust people who are non-conformists. The organisation cannot trust the individual, the individual must trust the organisation.'

This book also says that a single fast-food hamburger can contain meat from hundreds of cattle which spend their last days packed in feed lots full of pools of manure. The author quotes a study which concluded that poor hygiene in meat production means that there are more faecal bacteria in the average American kitchen sink than on the average American lavatory seat.

And it's certainly not confined to America. When I saw that McDonald's had invaded the beautiful, magical old city of Venice I realised that we had seen the end of civilisation as we once knew it. I'm with Kelly Brownell on this: our food environment is toxic.

The Emotional Component

To the already complex web of interrelated causes of fatness must be added one of the most potent factors: the emotional component.

Eating is comforting. Most people at some time, on some occasions or in some circumstances eat for comfort. Eating is nice, when other things in life are giving us trouble. When we feel empty in a psychic sense, a full stomach can help. Eating can blunt fear, pain and worry. People who are unhappy or disturbed eat to 'stuff down their emotions'.

This is not a metaphor or, at least, not simply a metaphor. When you are in distress of any kind your body knows there is a good drug it can get hold of for you and it is to be found in food: specifically, in carbohydrate. When people eat for emotional reasons they are unlikely to crave a pork chop. Carbohydrate will be the food of choice and combined with fat it is particularly palatable, hence the widespread appeal of chocolate. When you eat these things, your brain releases serotonin, the feel-good chemical. Your problems don't go away; the feelings associated with them are still with you but somehow you can bear them more easily than if you had not eaten.

Sceptics will say that many, many people have difficult childhoods and severe problems but they don't all stuff themselves and get fat. Of course not everyone does this. It depends on your physical and emotional make-up (the genetically predisposed fat person is more likely to turn to food), and on what food meant to you as a child. Children are rewarded with nice things to eat when they are good or on special occasions. They are comforted with food (a sweet when they fall over). And parents sometimes give food to assuage their guilt about something that they know they are failing to provide. Emotional eating usually has deep roots. A childhood of neglect, loneliness, fear or abuse will often be at the bottom of severely disordered, emotionally driven eating in adulthood.

Jill Welbourne cites as an example a cardiac technician she once worked with:

He was 15 stone, a perfectly normal weight for his height, he was bright, and he enjoyed his job. The surgeon he worked for retired and the new one thought that surgeons were God's gift and technicians were lower than the dust. He spent his time bullying, harassing and denigrating this chap who had nowhere else to go because he was at the top of his particular ladder. If the technician had been rude he would have lost his job so he spent each day stuffing down his anger, swallowing his bile and being compliant even when treated outrageously and made to look silly in front of his juniors. But he did it by swallowing doughnuts and chocolate and got to 21 stone. Then the nasty surgeon left and a third consultant came along. He was nice, treated the technician well and his weight returned to normal.

Weight problems are never about food before feelings. People need to look at the feeling roots first.

Diary of a Compulsive Eater

Karen is 38 and weighs just over 20 stone. Her life has been difficult but in no particularly dramatic way. Her parents divorced when she was six; her mother was a depressive who used alcohol to mask her pain. From childhood Karen used food to mask hers and would spend all her pocket money on chocolate.

Life was reasonably comfortable and Karen was bright. She trained as a teacher and worked until her first child was born when she was 29. Now with two children, she herself has been divorced and has married again. She would like to go back to work but does not think she would get a teaching job at her weight and is too afraid to try. She feels she could not face the rejection.

Karen sees her life as a series of rejections. She has never felt good enough. She thinks people will always want to leave her because she is lacking in some essential quality. She thinks it is only a matter of time before her husband Keith 'sees through' her and leaves too.

I first met Karen after she wrote to me on the publication of my first book.[8] She wanted to come and see me to talk about the issues raised in the book. I liked her a lot and I found her children delightful: a reflection of good mothering in difficult circumstances. We have stayed in touch and in the years I have known her, Karen's weight has steadily climbed.

She is unhappy and she deals with her feelings by eating. She has great insight into her problem and knows she is her own worst enemy, but she does not know how to befriend herself and is a little suspicious of the motives of people who befriend her. As Groucho Marx said, she would not want to join any club that would accept her as a member.

Because she is concerned about the health risks of being so large, Karen asked her doctor for help. He referred her to the surgery dietitian and also arranged for a few sessions with the practice counsellor. The dietitian simply gave her factual information that she already had. The counsellor recognised a deep-rooted problem but was not able in six sessions to do more than skim the surface.

Karen desperately wants to lose weight: she fears that she will die before her children grow up. She knows what her problem is. She knows that all she has to do is eat less – as if it were that simple – but she just cannot. At this moment, weight loss for Karen is not an option. Her relationship with food is so complex, her drive to eat is so powerful that unless she can get to the roots of the emotions behind it, she will not be able to lose weight. When she knew I was writing this book, she asked me to include her story.

Karen is now paying to see a counsellor privately. She has been asked to keep a food and feelings diary. What follows is an extract, a week in the pattern of Karen's life:

1 January

Breakfast: Toast and marmalade, tea. Feel okay.

10 a.m.: Tired. Want to eat for no discernible reason. Ate six bourbon biscuits, don't even like them but couldn't stop.

11 a.m.: Keith [husband] came in and wanted elevenses. Gave him mince pies and ate two. Felt out of control but what the hell.

Lunch: Had to stop myself eating more than I needed. Am feeling constantly anxious, apprehensive. Want to *stuff myself full*.

4.30 p.m.: Jan arrived bringing chocolates. Why? Can't she see I've got a problem? She opened them and offered them round. I took one, then when she and K weren't looking I took another – and ended up eating five. So ashamed – tried to cover the gaps with papers but she and K will see how many are missing. Mince pies for tea. Then sneaked more chocolates. Feel so dirty.

Supper: Had seconds. Didn't need it. Had chocolate pudding, gave myself a bigger piece than the others, though broke it up a bit so they wouldn't notice. I hope.

2 January
Breakfast: Okay but then finished the chocolates when the

others weren't looking. So surreptitious and sly. Too much food around, am drawn like a magnet. Keep nibbling but *can't stop.* *What is this all about?*

Lunch: Bread and cheese, normal amount. A sense of control! Wish Jan wasn't staying. She's getting on my nerves with her carping. Felt like snapping at her. Ate biscuits instead.

Tea: Christmas cake. Want to keep eating and eating but cannot analyse the craving. *Need.*

Supper: Okay. Jan gone thank God. But I'd eaten biscuits before supper. We finished the chocolate pudding and I hoped K would leave his but he didn't. Disappointed and relieved but more disappointed.

3 January
Breakfast is always okay. Nothing to record.

10 a.m.: Banana, satsumas, sneaked more biscuits. Am afraid K will notice. Feel hugely fat and imagine I have put on a stone in three days.

Lunch: Normal. So tired. Slept, horrible fantasy dream that my body was too big for my bed.

Tea: Cheese sandwich. Can't stop nibbling. Too much cheese *with* it, not even just in it. When I cut cheese it's in my mouth before I can stop it. It's a battle to get it on the bread.

Supper: Normal, though there were potatoes left in the dish and I compulsively gobbled them up while pretending to throw them away.

4 January
Breakfast. Okay.

11 a.m.: Intended to have a banana but saw stale Battenburg cake. Hate Battenburg. Gobbled it up – sweet and horrible. Why did I eat it? What did it do? Felt gross, grotesque.

Lunch: One and a half sandwiches. Ate slowly and felt anxious that it wasn't enough. Am I discerning a distinction between physical and emotional hunger? I only know I need to eat a lot because if I don't I feel the most incredible anxiety and yearning. But I don't know what it's about. B [counsellor] says food takes the edge off feelings and saves me having to experience them. I don't know about that. I certainly am aware of great emotional pain. Do I supress it with food? Odd idea.

1.30 p.m.: Only an hour since lunch but spotted a packet of bacon crisps that someone had left around. *Why do I eat these things when all I feel afterwards is guilt and disgust?* Come to think of it, I feel those things even when eating so I gobble very fast to get it over with. No enjoyment. Just feels necessary.

2 p.m.: I am full. I don't need anything till 5. Let's see if I can wait until then and perhaps reward myself with something nice.

3 p.m.: Ate two apples. They were in the bowl so I ate them.

5 p.m.: Do I deserve my treat? Had it anyway – two crumpets with butter.

Supper: Okay.

11 p.m.: Ate banana I didn't need.

5 January
Breakfast.

11.30 a.m.: Too hungry. Banana. I dreamt last night that there were chocolate biscuits still in the tin. I thought they'd all gone but I looked and there were two! Ate them of course. Would have eaten 10 if they'd been there. How must it feel to eat like a normal person?

Lunch: I actually felt full and didn't need lunch but couldn't not eat it. Tried to leave some but couldn't. Why?

5 p.m.: Two crumpets with jam.

6 p.m.: Supper is going to be late so had bread and cheese. Very anxious that supper might not be ready in time (in time for what?).

Supper: Okay.

Midnight: Putting remains of meal away in fridge I had a spoonful

– then another till I'd finished it. Why, oh why? It was much better when I was anorexic but I don't know how to do that now.

6 January
Breakfast: Okay.

Lunch: Too much. I feel so disgusted. Very flat, tired. I cannot bear this hugeness any more. I keep thinking that I will burst out of my skin. I have such stretch marks – what if they give way?

6 p.m.: Bread and jam.

8 p.m.: Five satsumas. Failed again.

9 p.m.: Supper and then a huge Danish pastry left over from Keith's lunch. Felt so disgusted. Realise that I only know about almost total denial or overeating. Food is like a drug. It would be better not to eat at all.

7 January
Breakfast: Okay. Why is this meal always okay? It's normal. It all goes wrong after that.

11 a.m.: Banana. Good! Not hungry after it.

12.30 p.m.: Why does any sense of control always end in my downfall? Made huge curry for lunch and when it was cooked I stood spooning it out of the saucepan and down my throat. Then I gave myself a large bowl of it for lunch. Felt utterly numb. This is never going to stop.

Later: Went to put curry (some left) in freezer but couldn't without eating a whole lot more. Thought about why. Realised that when I am exposed to nice, normal foods, as opposed to the one Ryvita and one apple I allowed myself when I was anorexic, I feel deprived if I don't eat too much.

8 January
Breakfast: Okay.

11 a.m.: One satsuma – hey, this is great!

1.30 p.m. Four people for lunch. They brought me chocolates. Ate normally till they left then fell on the chocs. Only managed to stop by throwing them into the flower bed. Immediately wanted to go and get them so went out and stomped them into the earth. I am a mountain – a monster.

Appointment with B: She has given me a problem to solve – how to get what I need without trying to get it through food. But I don't feel I need anything but food though rationally I *know* I don't need all this rubbish I eat. It occurs to me reading through this that all my feelings are about how I feel about food and eating. I don't seem to express many other kinds of emotions. All my energy is taken up with guilt and self-disgust about food while at the same time longing for it.

Karen has decided to give counselling six months and if by then she is not on the way to solving her eating problem she will be referred for surgery. I am not a qualified psychologist so I cannot analyse her diary, but it sounds very much as though she is dealing with two conflicting problems. There is the emotionally driven craving to eat and there is also the famine response. Karen has been on several severe low-calorie diets in the past and there is a sense of panic about her eating pattern. Even when she knows she is full and can last a few hours, within a short time she is eating again. The body's need to fill itself with as much as possible whenever possible comes from the experience of severe deprivation; this, combined with Karen's need for food to suppress feelings, makes a potent mix.

What makes me so angry is that Karen is not receiving help from the medical profession. She is seeing a counsellor but she is having to pay and can ill afford it. She thinks the counsellor is good but without much experience of eating disorders. Compulsive eating is an eating disorder in the same spectrum as anorexia and bulimia nervosa.

But people are not fascinated by fat in the way they are by anorexia. Look at the attention received by the late Princess Diana when she presented a tragic picture with her anorexia and bulimia; she evoked public and press sympathy and had a high-profile eating disorders therapist. On the other hand, the Duchess of York, who constantly gained and lost weight, was treated with scorn and jeers and dubbed the Duchess of Pork. A psychologist who works in an eating disorders clinic privately told me that fat people don't get a look in because the academics who head the clinics don't find fatness of much interest. Certainly resources are stretched and there have to be quotas, but they are not stretched evenly.

Fat people are supposed to do it by themselves. When you consider the complex causes of obesity – the genetic and emotional components combined with the havoc wreaked on the body by low-calorie dieting – it should make you see red. The body police in the government and the medical profession thunder on about the health risks and the cost to the nation of obesity but provide precious little in the way of resources to help people combat it. There are only eight obesity clinics in Britain and they have long waiting lists.

If it is true, as they would have us believe, that the health risks of obesity are considerable, why are they not funding clinics and practitioners to help those people who cannot lose weight? I have been told that the reason anorexics receive treatment is that their lives are in danger. But so, we are told, are ours! They can't have it both ways.

Some Rare Causes

There are other, relatively rare reasons for overweight. Prader Willi syndrome is a horrific, complex illness where sufferers feel hungry all the time and just cannot stop eating. Cushing's Disease makes people very fat. Polycystic ovary syndrome also causes considerable weight gain. Certain drugs, notably steroids, make people put on large amounts of weight. There is still much that is not known about the effects of disease, drugs and hormones on body weight.

What we do know is that overweight and obesity are perhaps more complicated than any other human condition. There is no single known cause and no cure. There are ways of losing weight but I know from experience that there will always be that fat person struggling to get out again.

Eating Is a Complex Issue

For some people, permanent weight loss is not an option. For physical and/or psychological reasons – such as lack of the satiety hormone, leptin – some will not be able to cut their energy intake and increase their output sufficiently to enable their bodies to reduce themselves in size. Others will *need* to eat for emotional reasons. As Julian Barth put it: 'In some people the impulses to eat *cannot* be overridden.'[9]

What is certain is that those individuals who weigh upwards of 40, 50, even 60 stone, and who suffer unimaginable physical and emotional pain, have not wilfully reached that state. The causes of such obesity are too complex to allow for censure.

Eating behaviour is rarely a question of having three balanced, calorie-appropriate meals a day. Just as there is a great diversity of size, so there is in the way people eat. There are large people who claim to eat like a mouse and thin people who gorge themselves without gaining weight. There are fat people who eat like gourmands and thin people who eat just enough to live. There are both large and 'normal'-weight people who don't think of quantity or calories or dieting, but who maintain a stable weight.

And there are those who eat to excess but never show it on their bodies: the bulimics, and those who repeatedly gain and lose the same half stone or so. The reasons for being fat are far more complex than can be summed up in a simple assessment of a person's eating behaviour.

Chapter Five
Seven Irrefutable, Unarguable Reasons Why You Should Not Lose Weight

My Doctor Says I Should Lose Weight

Most doctors will tell you that you have no good reason not to lose weight. The only reason in their mind for you to stay the size you are is if that size happens to be a 10. I think it is the other way round: doctors should give you a very good reason why you *should* lose weight. And having done so, they should back it up with sound factual evidence. They are not gods and we do not have to take their word on trust, especially where weight is concerned. Several studies have shown doctors to be among the most prejudiced of people, considering their large patients to be weak-willed, ill-disciplined, slovenly, lazy and greedy.[1]

There are, of course, exceptions. I collect them because they are rare and I offer them to you now. Dr Jill Welbourne, oft quoted in this book, is one. She is in the rather unusual position of being a doctor who is nagged by doctors to lose weight. She silences them with one word: 'Evidence?' The majority of her patients have been anorexic or bulimic: in other words, obsessed with becoming or remaining thin. Her success rate with them has been splendid, suggesting that rather than being afraid that if they followed her advice they might end up large like her, Jill's patients respond constructively to her motherly concern and sound good sense.

Dr Carole Rushford, my own GP, is another, proving that her patients' physical, mental or emotional problems do not require their weight to be taken into her assessment of them unless they request that it be so.

Not only is Carole Rushford completely non-judgmental, she has also managed to refer me to consultants who are not weight prejudiced. When I suffered from apparently intractable endometrial hyperplasia, Carole sent me to Mr Ken Bidgood, a gynaecologist, assuring me that he was one of the good guys. He was, in every sense. The treatment for the condition is usually hysterectomy. Forty years of brainwashing had convinced me that if I had surgery I would die. I was fat, therefore I was a 'surgeon's nightmare' and 'a grave anaesthetic risk'.

Ken Bidgood was having none of that. His core belief is that you treat each patient according to her needs; he gives equal treament to everyone. He doesn't judge them on their size or the fact that they smoke or drink or behave in any way considered socially unacceptable. He is passionately opposed to prejudice and says that he cringes when he hears some of the remarks made by his colleagues about large patients.

He said that he would not have a problem operating on me. He told me of a woman of about 18 stone on whom he had performed a hysterectomy the day before. It took two people instead of one to do the operation, and it took an hour and a half instead of the usual twenty minutes. 'But so what?' he said. He does not deny that there can be difficulties: 'Holding back eight inches of adipose tissue is not easy', and adds that sometimes it is difficult to ventilate very large patients. But he does not make weight loss a condition of treatment.

Ken went a long way towards undoing some of the damage inflicted on me by the medical profession but their prophecies of doom had sunk too deep into my psyche. I was still afraid to have an operation. We talked it through. The anaesthetic was my biggest fear. So he offered to do it under epidural. When I told him that I was still reluctant, he said that he completely respected my feelings. The danger with endometrial hyperplasia is that it is a pre-cancerous condition which makes hysterectomy the safest option. So I had a biopsy every year in order to keep an eye on the state of my endometrium. Several years later, it seems to have returned to normal.

During the course of those years I came to know Ken Bidgood quite well. More than once we discussed his attitude to seriously overweight patients and I realised that people really are all equal in his sight. When you live in a prejudiced world, one where medical prejudice is perhaps the sternest of all, it is an eye opener to hear the views of a practitioner who says 'This patient is overweight. So what?' This man accorded me a dignity rarely permitted when medicine and overweight collide.

Jill Welbourne, an anaesthetist before she specialised in eating disorders, is of the same mind. 'It is not more dangerous giving an anaesthetic to an overweight person,' she avers. 'It is just more difficult and doctors don't like hard work. It's the difference between reading a Mills and Boon and a Dickens.'

I have recently encountered Dr Julian Barth, who runs an obesity clinic at Leeds General Infirmary. He is cynical about the reasons for refusing to provide medical treatment to the overweight, and for making weight loss a condition of treatment. He also strongly believes that the accusation of overeating is pejorative. In addition to these golden qualities, he's also jolly nice to talk to. Add him to your list of rare medical discoveries.

Then there's Dr Peter Nixon, a consultant cardiologist – though, sadly, he's retired. That's five humanitarian, non-judgmental doctors of great integrity, none of whom make weight loss a condition of treatment. If I can collect five, there must be more, but you have to seek them out.

It is essential to have a GP you can trust not to bang on about weight. The only way to find one is to go and interview them. This is a bit tedious since in order to make an appointment you have to register. You can do so as a temporary resident which just means filling in a form each time you see a different doctor. They will probably be slightly taken aback that you have come to give them the once over, but they'll get over it. You don't need to take up much of their time; all you need to do is ask them if your weight is going to be an issue, if it is going to affect their assessment or treatment of you. You should ask them if they are going to want you to lose weight. You will get a clear idea straight away as to whether this is going to present a problem. I had a couple of very polite interviews with doctors, during which there was mutual agreement that we would not suit each other (at the time I had no intention of ever trying to lose weight again). If the doctor is not right for you, try again until you find one you feel comfortable with.

I have discovered that most people react with trepidation to the idea of interviewing doctors because most of us are afraid of them. They are the only authority figures to have retained a godlike status in the eyes of the laity. While the clergy, the legal profession, politicians and royalty no longer command respect simply on account of who they are, the medical profession – notwithstanding its blunders, its frequent callousness, its high rate of alcoholism and its Harold Shipmans – is still regarded with a kind of awe that drives me mad with frustration. It is because they have so much power: the power of life and death. At some level of consciousness we fear that if we cross them they may withhold treatment – maybe only by default, not deliberate decision – but it's a risk we feel we cannot afford to take. They also have the power to remove us from their list without an explanation. Best to keep on the right side of them, we think, and not risk doing anything that might upset that balance of power. And so they go on behaving like gods because we treat them like gods.

If you want to find a doctor who will not discriminate against you because you are fat, you do not have to threaten them. You don't have to be defiant or defensive about it. You just need to be very quiet and dignified and have your questions prepared beforehand. It is an entirely reasonable thing to do. You may find it helpful to take along the SIZE rights charter (available from SIZE, see Resources). Under 'Positive Health Care' the charter asks for: 'The right to informed, specialised health care, focused on attaining disease prevention and optimum good health regardless of size. An end to weight-loss treatments, drugs and surgery which cannot prove their long-term effectiveness and safety.'

I feel very strongly about the importance of creating awareness in the medical profession. They have minimum training in communication and empathy. Several doctors have confessed to me that they were actually taught in medical school to be nasty to fat people so that they would be shamed into losing weight. If you receive a fattist comment from a doctor you need to point it out. Pleasantly. In a non-confrontational way.

By one of those little quirks of synchronicity I had to make a fairly sudden visit to a GP in the middle of writing this section. Having just undertaken an 11-hour train journey, I developed quite severe pain in my calf. Mindful of the possibility of deep vein thrombosis, especially as it killed my mother, I rang the NHS Direct Line, a service I can thoroughly recommend. There is something liberating about being able to discuss a health matter without feeling that the practitioner is probably taking your weight into account.

The nurse I spoke to said that several factors were troubling her and that I should see a doctor immediately. I could not get a same-day appointment with my own GP, so had to see another in the practice. I felt uneasy; most of us who have suffered from fat threats, taunts or ill-concealed disgust on the part of doctors are fairly nervous about seeing one we have not met. This GP examined my leg and said he did not think it was a thrombosis. That was all I required. He then said 'Your weight doesn't help, of course.' Apart from the fact that this remark was quite gratuitous, it did not make sense. Having told me that I had no thrombosis, what *was* it that my weight did not help? It was just the usual doctors' reaction to an overweight patient. He then asked me a perfunctory question about what I had been doing in the past few days. I said I had been on holiday where I had done a great deal of walking. 'You're probably not used to so much walking', he said patronisingly.

Normally, I would have tried to pluck up the courage to challenge him on these remarks, but he had been called out, his surgery was running very late and I knew he would not be receptive. So I wrote to him the next day. The following is part of the letter:

Dear Dr X,

I came to see you yesterday about a painful leg which was causing me some concern as I had just undertaken a very long train journey. You were able to reassure me that there was no thrombosis and I would like to thank you for your time and trouble.

During the consultation you made reference to my weight. I found this completely gratuitous; that was not the reason for consulting you. I don't know if you are aware of the studies that show doctors to be one of the most weight-prejudiced groups in society? It is an alarming fact that many overweight people are reluctant to go to their GPs because they know they will be nagged about their weight at a time when they are feeling vulnerable or frightened. I have known of people with potentially life-threatening conditions, such as breast lumps, who have put off seeing the doctor because they cannot face a lecture about obesity.

It has not escaped my attention that I am overweight and pointing it out does not help. I am aware that for many, chiding patients about their weight is in the nature of a medical knee-jerk reaction. We, who are overweight, know we are. Every day we receive messages from all around us that we are basically Bad People. We really don't need it underlined by our doctors.

I'm writing this, not to complain, but to say please think before you refer to a patient's weight. You can be entirely constructive without saying the obvious: 'Your weight doesn't help.'

Yours sincerely,

SCB

I didn't get a reply. Now does that suggest the doctor felt guilty or that he believed my complaint was beneath contempt: (a) because he thought that size-related offensiveness was an oxymoron, or (b) because the complaint was made by a fat woman and therefore invalid?

More often than not, doctors want to control fat people in the only way they think appropriate: by making them lose weight. And if you don't – well, it's *your* fault, of course, as Lee Kennedy found during her desperate attempts to become thinner.

The consultant then insisted I go on a proper measure-everything-out-count-how-many-strands-of-pasta-type regime. I know most certainly that I can't stick to that sort of thing (who could, for life?). He waspishly dismissed me as being immature and said I'd have no success until I changed my 'chaotic' lifestyle! In passing I'd just like to mention I find it curious that doctors specialising in obesity are *always* (in my experience) little birdlike, bespectacled men with quaint views on 'lifestyle' and sexuality.

Many doctors make no effort to control their contempt for the overweight. Dr Thomas Stuttaford, regular medical columnist in *The Times*, dishes out the tired old stereotypes. 'Obesity leads to such conditions as sweating and snoring,' he pronounces.[2] So what's happened to my glands, then? I never sweat. (Of course, we know that thin people never snore nor sweat.) And did you know that 'In fashionable hotels and health clubs, the overweight can be seen struggling across a width of the pool before rewarding their exertions with delicious cakes and cream.'[3] What a boring, unoriginal thing to say. And come to think of it, in his photo he does look birdlike and bespectacled.

The point is that doctors cannot have it both ways. They can't mock and rubbish the overweight *and* pretend to be concerned about related health issues. We just don't believe them.

No movement for change can get off the ground until we make our oppressors aware of what they are doing. Doctors won't change their attitudes unless we continue to educate them.

I Must Lose Weight or My Health Will Suffer

To say that concern about health is not a good reason to lose weight sounds like heresy so I must qualify this particular heading.

I do not propose here to discuss in detail the controversy about weight and health since I have already done so in a previous book.[4] All I will say is that the evidence for a connection between overweight and poor health is extremely conflicting. There are literally thousands of studies on the health risks of overweight and obesity: so many that for every one you read, you can find another that will diametrically oppose and apparently disprove it. When you read the research your head starts to whirl like that of the girl in the film *The Exorcist*.

The author Charles Roy Schroeder, in his excellent book *Fat Is Not a Four-Letter Word*, calls research 'a tainted deity'.[5]

> False and misleading results of research occur even in studies conducted by the brightest and most ethical of scientists. Because there is such pressure to publish in order to advance – relative to salaries, promotions, professional status, and to acquire research grants – some scientists rush through research, make errors, and publish prematurely.

There is so much fraud in research, says Shroeder, that it has been given its own name: 'lab-scam'.

Of course, there are health risks to being severely overweight. Not even the most militant size-acceptance activist will claim that a 400-pound individual is not at some risk. But then so are the very thin (I am excluding thinness caused by existing sickness). So are those who drink alcohol, drive cars and participate in sport. No one is suggesting that they give up those activities; indeed they are positively encouraged. Alcohol and sport in particular are said to be good for us even though they cost the NHS millions; driving a car is a fact of modern life.

What does seem to be clear is the health risk of repeated dieting.[6] This is why I have suggested that losing weight to improve health is not in itself a good reason. It is not enough. The motivation to lose weight has to be very strong indeed for it to be successful. You should only embark on a diet because you really really *want* to, not because you feel you ought to. Not even because your health would improve if you did. Losing weight is so difficult that you have to be 100 per cent gung-ho about it. If you are not, you will certainly regain the weight and your health will be the worse for it. Then you may decide to try again . . . and you're on the yo-yo route.

Of course, you could feel strongly enough *because* your health means so much to you. Some health problems, like arthritis, are greatly exacerbated by extra weight and weight loss can bring noticeable relief.

This was the case for my friend Pamela (the one who did not believe size prejudice existed), whose arthritis grew worse as she got heavier. In intense pain and only able to walk a few steps with difficulty and with a crutch, she embarked on a diet – a good one, no low-calorie rubbish – about six months ago.

But Pamela did not want to lose weight; she has no problem with being fat. She tried the diet for the sake of her health. As her heart was not in it, she lost only a few pounds and then quickly regained them. Although her eating plan was balanced and she did not experience hunger, she missed the rich food she loves. This is what she said at the point when she was trying to decide what to do:

I find it difficult to impose restrictions on my eating – not so much the amount but rather the type of food. I love Chinese and Indian, meat of all kinds and chocolate – who doesn't? What do I intend to do about this state of affairs? Do I care enough to undertake a diet for the rest of my life and give up the food I love? This decision has been a huge battle for me and I am still not certain I have won. Or that I really want to. My health is at stake and that is the biggest reason to change. The social pressures are of less interest to me as I believe my personality and ability will see me through. Perhaps I am storing up terrible trouble for myself. If only I had a crystal ball . . .

A few months after that, Pamela realised that she did not have sufficient enthusiasm for losing weight. She made a conscious decision to remain at her present weight even though the loss of a few pounds did seem to alleviate her arthritic pain a little. She said 'I would rather be in pain than go without the foods I love.' That is a brave admission and I believe she should be supported in her decision.

Her health is further complicated by high blood pressure, high cholesterol levels and diabetes. She knows that she may not live to a great age. But she is already 70, and apart from her disability she is in great good health with masses of energy and enthusiasm. The research on weight and health is not conclusive about premature death from overweight: too many other factors have to come into play. Pamela has good genes for longevity.

The other day I visited a 93-year-old lady. She has always been very large; she is bright, sharp, funny and fully present. She can't walk so easily now and she is in pain from arthritis – yet she confounds the prophets of doom. Fat people are not supposed to live to 93 but, believe me, she is not rare.

The doomsayers would probably say she'd live a lot longer if it were not for her weight! They'd wag their finger and say 'You'll never live to be 100, you know.'

People should never be bullied into losing weight for their health, nor scared into feeling they must 'do something about it' or they will die an early death. This kind of medical blackmail is totally unacceptable and very distasteful.

We must never lose sight of the truth hidden beneath the prejudice and that is that you can be very fat and very fit. Frances White, a former president of NAAFA, is a woman of high weight who knows that her prognosis is good; she has the genes for it.

I'm told I must be diabetic, I must have high blood pressure, I must have high cholesterol, etc, because I'm fat. I get tested. I return for the results and hear 'Oh, you're okay, don't worry.' I know I have none of these problems because they do not run in my family and I 'force' the doctor to read off the results so s/he must acknowledge that I have numbers a lot of thin people would kill for! I deeply resent that decisions are made about my health based on my size and these decisions are used to legitimise a bias against me on the job and in getting access to decent, compassionate care.

I had a blood test a little while ago. I asked the doctor – young, blonde, tall, slim, confident – who attended me if my cholesterol had been measured. I knew what she was thinking. She looked. 'It's lower than *mine*,' she said indignantly. It was a good moment!

The point about overweight and health is this: there *are* health risks at a very high weight and it would be foolish to discount them. But, based on the poor prognosis for permanent weight loss and the helplessness of the medical profession to improve this, the decision to stay a high but stable weight is a wise one if you know that you will probably regain any weight you lose.

What is more important is to maintain a stable weight and to maximise health and fitness whatever size you are. Professor Philip James of the International Obesity Task Force believes that simply maintaining weight is itself a major triumph. 'We are still obsessed with the idea of losing weight, yet to stop putting weight on is a staggering achievement.'[7]

My Husband/Partner/Boyfriend/Girlfriend/Mother Would Like Me to Be Slimmer

First ask a simple question. Ask it of this other person or of yourself, or ask it rhetorically, but *ask it*. Why? Why does this person, this *other*, want to alter *your* body? You may not get an honest answer, but there is a variety of reasons why someone of significance in your life may want you to lose weight.

Let's start off by giving people the benefit of the doubt. It could be out of genuine concern. In the minds of most people, medical or lay, it is written in stone that to be overweight is to be unhealthy. Even a tiny excess may shorten your life, say the pundits. Anyone who has not received this message has obviously been asleep for the last thirty years – or living in one of the increasingly few cultures where not only do they not believe this, but the nature of self-fulfilling prophecy sees to it that fat people are no less healthy than anyone else.

However, since most of us dwell in contemporary, health fascist society, we can expect that however intelligent our nearest and dearest, however informed about most aspects of modern life, the chances are they will have been duped over this particular one. They will be afraid that you are going to suffer from one of the dire, disabling fates of the fat and die an early death.

There are two things to consider here: the appropriate response of the non-fat and the appropriate response of the frankly fat. When I say non-fat I don't mean the size 14s. I mean the 16–18s, those women who are a stone or two over the weight they 'ought' (heavy inverted commas) to be. If you come into this category, inform your concerned loved ones that you are at no more risk than they are. Tell them that there is no evidence that at your size and weight there is anything to worry about healthwise. Tell them that on the contrary you actually have a better chance statistically of living longer than they do (if they are 'normal' weight). Quote the Norway study to them. This was the world's largest ever epidemiological study, which monitored 1.8 million participants over ten years. The lowest mortality rate was found to be amongst those who were approximately 30 per cent 'overweight'.[8]

The appropriate response of the frankly fat varies only in that there *are* some health risks at a high weight, but taking steps to maximise health cuts these risks considerably, as does losing just a small amount of weight. So reassure your beloveds. Give them research to read: Paul Ernsberger and Paul Haskew's *Rethinking Obesity* is an excellent overview of the academic research that shows dire predictions of early death to be exaggerated.[9] Get in touch with SIZE, which will provide all the necessary facts and support. If, after all this, they still express concern for your health be very suspicious. Pure prejudice often masquerades as concern. Any concern that takes the form of coercion or manipulation, however gently applied, is bogus. People have their own powerful agenda when weight is the issue and you need to see beyond what might be a mask.

Husbands and other partners may bring another kind of pressure to bear, one that is to do with *their* self-image. If you look at the newspaper ads for partners you will see that the word that appears constantly is 'slim'. In this context, where little information can be given in just a few lines, the word is synonymous with acceptable, normal. When used by the advertiser who is offering him or herself on the dating market, it says 'It's alright, you won't have to be ashamed of me.' When used by the one stating their requirements in a partner it means 'I won't go out with a fat person, whatever other qualities they may have.' Overweight people, looking for love, feel completely excluded from the dating agency/advertising game. They scan the ads in despair, seeing most of them requesting a 'slim' date. Sometimes, pathetically, you will see someone advertise themselves as 'pleasantly rounded', or 'plump, but dieting'.

Some dating agencies, especially the very expensive ones, will not take clients over a certain weight. When I met the proprietor of one such agency he said that he could not take money from large people (£3000 in this case) knowing that he wouldn't be able to provide them with a date. Oh sure, he knew that it was all wrong, that it was the person underneath that really counted but when you were looking for a soulmate, appearance was important. I did point out that soulmate and appearance were hardly compatible as terms of reference but he missed the point. Although I thought this man was a sleazebag, the fact is that he was right.

It's the old story: fatness equates all the negative qualities of greed, sloth and lack of discipline. If you choose a fat partner what is that saying about you? That you have no taste? That you couldn't get anything better? Or that those negative qualities, inseparable in so many people's minds with a fat body, are somehow implicit in you if your partner is overweight? This, sadly, is how the thinking runs.

When I appeared on an Esther Rantzen talk show about fatness and relationships, there were women there who had lost their husbands and partners because they (the women) had put on weight. One woman told a long story about being eight stone and happily married. She put on weight and 'ballooned' (the word tabloid reporters and women's magazines love) to 15 stone. Her husband left her as a consequence. So she did what any good wife should. She lost the weight and lo! he returned to her. She seemed entirely unaware of the fact that the bastard wasn't worth having and only wanted her if she boosted his image.

I wish I could say that this kind of behaviour only applied to men. But women impose the same shallow standards on their male partners and lesbians seem as culpable as anyone else. I remember being very shocked when I attended the first National Fat Women's Conference in 1989, and discovered that women can be as sizeist in their choice of female partners as I had always believed only men to be. And a lesbian friend of mine, who fell in love, was told by her *inamorata* that they could only start a relationship when my friend had lost two stone. Sad to say, she did have a bash at losing it although she soon came to her senses. There is only one kind of real love and that is unconditional.

Beware, too, the treachery of friends. Strike from your heart and your Christmas card list anyone who comes out with any variation of the following: 'Wouldn't you *feel* so much better if you lost weight?'; 'It's not that I mind that you're overweight, it's just that I care about your health.' (Possibly acceptable from a partner, not from a friend.); 'You've got such a pretty face...'; 'You *could* look so good.' I cannot count the number of times I have been on the receiving end of the first and the last of these highly loaded comments.

These remarks are prompted by anger and the need to control. The anger is about the constraints that women feel they are under; the fact that they are working damned hard to keep their own bodies in check and there you are letting it all hang out. They exercise iron control and they try to project that control onto their fatter friends. If they have to do it, why shouldn't you?

As Camryn Manheim points out in her autogiography *Wake Up, I'm Fat*,[10] whether or not we lose weight is our own business.

Next time you have an impulse to suggest that a friend or family member lose weight, take a minute to ask yourself why it is important enough to you to risk humiliating someone you care about to give this profound advice. Most people argue that they are merely looking out for the well-being of their loved ones, but I suggest that some other factor is at work here... Could it perhaps be embarrassment? Do we as a society just hate to be seen with fat people?

I find it impossible not to question the motives of those who would have us change. Nowhere is this more tellingly demonstrated than in the let-it-all-hang-out format of the confessional TV programme. There is a show on Britain's ITV channel called *Trisha*, which specialises in this sort of mass humiliation and seems to deal with the subject of fatness more often than anything else. One show, called 'I'm Fat and I'm Furious', produced the unfortunately named Grace, 'friend' of Maureen. Grace came on the set first and said that Maureen needed to lose weight because she wouldn't go out any more. This dialogue ensued:

Trisha: Have you told her this?
Grace: Not really, no
Trisha: Why not?
Grace: Because I don't want to hurt her feelings. I've never said to her 'Maureen, you look terrible, you need to lose weight.'

Enter Maureen stage left, tearful.

Trisha: Okay Grace, what do you want to say to Maureen?
Grace (turns to Maureen): You look gorgeous today but too overweight. It's ruining our friendship – not because I feel any different about you because I don't at all – but it's changing you. You don't want to go out, you don't want to do anything, you don't want to see anybody, you don't want to buy clothes...

Grace's reason for thus humiliating her friend was that Maureen had been 'very upset' about her weight. Her chief crime seems to have been not wanting to go out. When an audience member protested that it was personality that counted, Grace replied that Maureen was losing her personality.

Now Maureen, a rather sweet, vulnerable soul, professed gratitude to Grace. Maybe it all turned out well and they are closer than ever. Let's hope that Maureen is now going out.

Karen, a young mother on the same programme, was bullied by her own mother and told to lose weight. What I couldn't understand was that her mother looked about the same size as Karen, but it takes all sorts.

What I also can't understand is why people who say they can't go out because of their size (or for any other reason) are happy to appear on national television and say so!

One night, when I was a guest on a popular phone-in radio show, a woman rang to talk about her two friends. They were aged 43 and 45, she said, and not married because they were overweight. 'They have let themselves go,' she wailed. 'It drives me *mad* that they won't do anything about it.'

I was so amused by this that I wrote it down verbatim. The presenter of the show, Brian Hayes, had a reputation for bitter sarcasm and an acid tongue that could lacerate the boldest caller. I was very glad to leave the response to him!

Don't I Have a Moral and Social Obligation to Lose Weight? After All, I Am Taking up Too Much Space

Being fat is anarchic; it doesn't accord with the prescribed social order. A true anarchist will delight in her fatness and the size-acceptance movement has a good number of such people. They are saying 'I am fat. I have a right to be fat and to participate in everything in the same way as people who are of so-called normal weight. Society should accommodate me, I should not have to accommodate society.' These are the people who will ultimately change society's perception of fat people – if that ever happens.

You have the right to be the size you are, whatever that is. If there is a problem with physical space the answer is not to make fat bodies thinner, it is to create more space. There is a feminist theory that there is a patriarchal conspiracy to keep women thin because thinness equals powerlessness. Feminist columnist Suzanne Moore believes there is a simple formula: 'The more power women have in the world the less actual space we must occupy. Female bodies left to themselves are just unacceptable. They must be thoroughly controlled and the thinner you are the more control you are seen to have.'[11]

I do not see this as a feminist issue; I see it as one of social control. It is no easier nowadays to be a fat man than it is to be a fat woman. Thinness is the status quo but there is no good reason to aspire to this. Even though my personal choice has been to lose weight (though not in order to become a thin woman), my political stance is still 100 per cent anarchic.

It so happened that I reached my six-stone weight loss around the same time that Vanessa Feltz also lost the same amount, though mine was much slower. Unlike her, I hope I do not have the zeal of the convert. I do not think I am a better person, a more worthy person for losing weight. I did not feel any sense of obligation. It is, I think, both disingenuous and insulting to speak of fat people in 'them and us' terms. 'For every doughnut a fat person shoves down their cakehole, the rest of us are footing an astronomical bill,' she writes. She says she doesn't think anyone who is content to get stuck in turnstiles or take up two aeroplane seats should be made to change. But: 'Your body is the repository of your soul, and it's your responsibility to keep it in the most efficient working order you can. Responsibility is the operative word here. Responsibility to oneself, to one's family, to one's employer and ultimately, to society.'[12] This is a rallying cry, delivered with apparent satisfaction at her current body size. But there is a paradox here because the remarks she makes about fat people apply to the person she was and could easily become again.

If you lose weight because you believe you have a duty to conform, you are acceding to bullies. I know a woman who constantly complains that she does not have enough room in her seat on the London Underground because all too often she is sitting next to a fat person. She thinks they have a moral and social duty to lose weight – or keep out of the public arena. In fact she has said that fat people should stay at home because it is unpleasant for other people to have to look at them! Presumably there are times when she is seated next to someone less able, or with a lot of baggage or perhaps with a baby or small child on their lap, people who also take up more room than the meagre provision of an Underground train seat. I don't hear her complaining about those situations but that's because her aim is only the elimination of the fat.

There are *no* circumstances under which you have a moral or social obligation to lose weight. If you have an accident and it takes four paramedics to lift you onto a stretcher that is not your problem. If, in hospital, a nurse grumbles because she hurts her back lifting or moving you, *that* is not your problem. She should know how to lift and when to call for extra help. If she, with her training, does it wrong the responsibility for her backstrain is hers.

So forget any sense of compulsion or obligation. The idea that we have a moral duty to lose weight is a very persuasive one. But the kind of social control which seeks to reduce us all to weights that conform to the height/weight or BMI charts is really no different from Hitler's dream of the perfect race.

If I Lost Weight I Could Go Out and Buy a Whole New Wardrobe of Fashionable Clothes

There was a time when large people either had to have their clothes tailor-made for them or dress in the most hideous smocks and tents. I have an enduring memory of a fairly hideous seventies maroon polyester pinafore dress that bore the label 'Dee Dawson'. Yes, the children's eating disorders specialist was once a designer of clothes for large women. What a career change!

It was difficult in those days to find decent clothes if you were really large. Much of the time, I wore maternity dresses, even when I wasn't pregnant. Then came a chain called Evans Outsizes (now just called Evans). It was horrible walking into the shop, casting furtive glances around – a bit like going into a sex shop. Outsize is a particularly emotive word. Things have changed – not enough, but there are several good high-street chains for large women, a host of mail-order catalogues, including some good designer ones, and the range of sizes in non-specialist shops shows that manufacturers and retailers are beginning to heed the fashion needs of large women. I would say that any woman up to about size 24, of any age, could equip themselves with a decent wardrobe now. Beyond 24 the choice is more limited but it's still reasonable. Young women are not left out of this; some of the trendy high-street fashion chains are producing clothes in larger sizes and there is a mail-order catalogue exclusively for the young.

Losing weight in order to fit the fashions worn by the size 8–16s would almost certainly be a temporary state. Manners (may) maketh man but clothes definitely do not make woman. It isn't enough. If just the idea of a trendy wardrobe were to set you off on a weight-loss regime, then sadly you would probably find that next season your new clothes would no longer fit. Then, psychologically, you would feel like hell.

'They' say you should never keep clothes that are too small, waiting for the time you diet yourself back into them. I think this is probably fairly sound. When I was very large I did keep my favourite clothes in the attic, the ones I couldn't fit into any more. Every time I saw them I felt terrible pangs of regret and great surges of disgust and low self-worth. There was a great longing for that less fat woman I had been and it didn't do me any good. Eventually, I got rid of them. Of course, human nature being entirely perverse, I now wish I hadn't. There were lovely things that I *could* wear now – but, on the whole, I think chucking them was the right thing to do.

I have noticed that when 'normal'-sized women put on a little weight and go on a diet they often say it is because they have to, because they cannot fit into their clothes and they cannot afford to buy new ones. But when women lose weight, they can't wait to buy new, smaller ones. Suddenly a new wardrobe *is* affordable. But it's not a good reason to lose weight.

My Boss Wants Me to Lose Weight. S/he Says I Don't Present a Good Image of the Company

If your boss said he didn't think company image was enhanced by the fact that you were gay, of ethnic origin, walked with a crutch or were a working mother, you could take him to the Equal Opportunities Commission and thence to court and you would win. Unfortunately, he can say what he likes about your size with legal impunity.

There has been much debate about including size in the legislation against discrimination in the workplace but so far it has not happened in Britain, though size discrimination is illegal in some parts of America. Some acceptance activists do not want to see the law changed because they say that fatness should be seen as part of the normal spectrum of human size and not put into a special category of its own. While I see their point, sexual orientation, ability and all the other diversities of humankind are also part of the normal spectrum. If people who do not conform to the WASP heterosexual ideal can be protected by law so that they do not have to fear dismissal or discrimination in the workplace, then I believe this legislation should extend to people of size.

The National Size Acceptance Network (SIZE) is campaigning for fairness at work. Its charter demands: 'The right to equal opportunity in employment. Potential employees should be selected on the strength of their qualifications and ability to do the job, not on a potential employer's prejudice, aesthetic bias or insurance height–weight charts which are known to be misleading.'

I took part in one phone-in programme on fatness during which a man called to say that as a managing director he would never employ a fat person. They were slovenly, he said, they took more time off work, they got 'circulatory diseases'. Safe in the security of anonymity (only first names are asked for on these programmes), this man proceeded to roundly damn the overweight in the workforce.

A few days later, I received a call from a national tabloid. The reporter said they thought they had managed to track down this man and were about to 'out' him. They just wanted to hear my side of the story. He was, they said, the MD of a company belonging to a very large, high-profile group.

The piece appeared; the man was outed, complete with photo. The paper reported that he was going to live abroad. For once justice was seen to be done, even though some might have called it a kangaroo court. But in the absence of legislation what other protection is there for the overweight who are discriminated against?

In a survey carried out by the University of Michigan it was discovered that fat people find it more difficult to get a job in the first place, are less likely to get promotions, pay rises and other benefits and even lose jobs because of their weight.[13] The survey found that fat people are seen as lazy, sloppy and lower class. For every extra stone a woman carried, her salary dropped by more than 1.5 per cent.

Dr Andrew Hill of the Association for the Study of Obesity said 'There is no evidence to suggest fat people will be any less reliable or more slobbish than thin ones. Attacking someone because of their weight has become the last socially acceptable form of prejudice.'[14]

So what should you do if your boss wants you to lose weight and you know your job is not protected by anti-sizeist legislation? Well, you *are* protected from unfair dismissal and being fat is not enough in itself to get you fired. But that is only part of the problem. If you suspect you are being denied opportunities because of your size, then take control. Face your boss with it. Tell him or her what your feelings are. If your boss has not actually said that it is your weight that is the issue, and if you tackle him or her in a non-confrontational way, you will discover one of two things. Either that you were mistaken (paranoia is not uncommon in the overweight but just because you're paranoid it doesn't mean they're *not* out to get you!); or that your employer has no issue with your weight and that perhaps there is a problem with another aspect of the way you do your job – or that s/he is indeed prejudiced in which case you can either try re-educating this person (it can be surprising how receptive people can be and how ignorant they are of their own subconscious prejudice); you can stick it out; or you can leave.

The one thing you should never do is allow yourself to be cajoled or bullied by your employer into losing weight.

But I'm Costing the Country Millions

In February 2001, the National Audit Office (NAO) produced a long-awaited report, *Estimating the Cost of Obesity in England*, which of course excited great media attention (sound of baying hounds – another chance to savage the fatties). This computed the direct cost of treating obesity: visits to doctor or hospital, drugs, surgery specifically for obesity. Then there was the cost of treating the consequences of obesity: all those illnesses we're supposed to get. Then they accounted for earnings lost due to premature mortality and earnings lost due to sickness absence.

The report concluded that fat people were costing the country £2.6 billion. Of that sum, £9.5 million was said to be spent on treating obesity itself; £469.9 million on the consequences of obesity and a staggering £2.5 billion on lost earnings.

The methodology used to compile this report is extremely suspect. The NAO estimated the costs by 'taking a prevalence-based, cost-of-illness approach based on extensive literature review and relying on published primary data'. My hackles were up already.

The costs of obesity treatments were assessed with relative ease: the cost of consultations with GPs, hospital admissions and outpatient attendances and the cost of drugs for weight loss. All of these were related to patients who had asked for medical help or treatment to reduce their weight.

Then the report put forward the alleged cost of treating the consequences of obesity. This covered 'diseases such as coronary heart disease which *can* [my italics] be directly attributed to obesity'. Not diseases that are attributable, just those that can be. They reviewed the literature for diseases which '*in theory* [my italics] would be eliminated if obesity were eliminated'.

In theory, note. So we can assume, can we not, that the costs they are talking about are only those which *in theory* could be attributed to obesity? They are not fact.

In searching for literature, they selected only 17 studies out of 3537 from which to extrapolate their data. The report announces casually that as there were limited data available from the UK, most of the data used were taken from international sources, especially from the United States.

But we are not Americans. Our lifestyle has not yet become Americanised. And the report has to acknowledge this. 'While the extent to which the same relative risks apply to the English population is uncertain, they nevertheless represent the best data available on which to base relative risk estimates.'

You see? Words like 'can' rather than the definite 'are'; phrases like 'in theory'; and now the admission that the extent to which the risks apply is 'uncertain'.

I smell a large colony of rats.

As for the earnings lost due to premature mortality, well, it's kind of the government to be so concerned about the individual, but you know, these poor people don't actually care that they're not earning any more because, you see, they've gone to 'a better place'. Perhaps the concern is for families? Admirable.

But all these fat people popping off early will help with the vexed problem of unemployment and save a bit of money there, won't it? Not just that, think of what the country will save in *pensions*! Just imagine if all the fat people lived as long as all the thin people – how much would that cost with them all working until 65, selfishly not leaving opportunities open for the unemployed, and corpulent nonagenarians bankrupting the country with their relentless weekly pension drawing?

As for loss of productivity and sickness benefits – well, how do they know it's the fat people? These are estimated on claims for benefit. So when you are ill and claim sickness benefit do you say 'Hello. Don't forget to register the fact that I am a Fat Person.'?

If I go to a doctor and am found to have high blood pressure (I haven't but it can happen to anyone), it will be attributed to my weight. No other cause will be sought. A *de facto* conclusion will be drawn. If my thin friend, same age, goes and is also found to have high blood pressure, they will enquire into her lifestyle, her diet, her family history. (Of my five friends who have high blood pressure requiring medication only one could be said to be overweight.) High blood pressure, type 2 diabetes and some forms of heart disease are more prevalent in the overweight but it is not as conclusive as that. Just because you are overweight does not mean you have heart disease, in the same way that just because you have heart disease does not mean you are overweight.

It's like those maths problems at school. 'A is fat and does not have heart disease. B is thin and does have heart disease. C is thin and does not have heart disease. Which kinds of people, fat or thin, get heart disease?' Or something like that. I never could do those problems.

There is no real proof of the extent of the incidence of so-called fatness-related diseases because there are so many variables. Deb Burgard, an American fat activist and fitness instructor, moderates a group called Show Me the Data, which is composed of activists, nutritionists and therapists. The group's slogan is 'correlation not causation'.[15]

'In this country,' says Frances White of NAAFA, 'fat people are constantly bombarded with a bogus statistic that says 300,000 fat people die in the US every year because of obesity. The real study, by a researcher named McGinnis, dates from 1993 and says 300,000 Americans die each year from lack of exercise and poor nutrition. We know fat folks who exercise live longer than thin people who don't exercise.'[16]

On the day the report came out I articulated my scepticism in a television interview. 'How can you be so *irresponsible*?' demanded the presenter in tones of the highest dudgeon. Why do people just believe these numbers without intelligent thought or any degree of analysis?

People love an excuse to have a go at the fat people. What about the cost of sports injuries? Smoking? DIY accidents? Alcohol-related illness *and* injury and death caused to others through drinking? I'm sure there are statistics on these and many other things. They just don't hit the headlines and make good people feel bad.

I strongly believe that the decision to lose weight *must* come from a position of unbiased, uninfluenced, personal choice. Whatever the reason for wanting to be thinner – social, psychological, emotional or health-based – it must be *yours*. If it is founded on coercion it is unacceptable in human rights terms. You should not feel that you have to conform to some prescribed medical, social or aesthetic standard.

Chapter Six
A Personal Odyssey

Childhood – and the Comfort of Food

I was a thin child with a slim mother and until the age of 11 I
didn't know the meaning of the words 'weight problem'. Puberty,
loneliness and the ready availability of chocolate and doughnuts
changed that. I grew up in a pub and my parents sold chocolate. I
can see it now in the stockroom: cardboard boxes full of bars of
Cadbury's Dairy Milk and Fruit and Nut. The stockroom was
next to the door to the stairs – which was next to the door I most
hated, the one that separated our living quarters from the bar. I
would come down in the evenings, wanting my mother to spend
some time with me. I'd open the door a crack and try to attract her
attention, but she was always frantic, rushing hither and thither
dispensing pints and gin and tonics and snowballs to the hordes
on the other side of the counter who clamoured for immediate
service. Life in a pub is hectic and my poor mother really did not
have the time to stop and attend to me. So I'd shut the door again
and sidle into the stockroom. I couldn't resist the siren call of
those purple-wrapped bars: my first experience of comfort eating.

The doughnuts were a treat, bought for me by my mother, who
lived with a constant, corrosive guilt that I only fully understood
after her premature death. She could not spend much time with
me but she could give me tempting things to eat. Looking back I
see that we ate very healthily. She was a good plain cook – but
healthy food is not special to a child. So my mother did what so
many mothers do: gave me something nice to stop the pain. Our
village bakery made the most incredibly delicious doughnuts –
soft, squidgy, full of jam. They were so *sensual*. Food like chocolate
and doughnuts is as much, if not more, about sensation than taste.
And so I grew plump. It wasn't entirely due to the wicked foods;
if it had been it would have happened earlier but I remained thin
until pubescent hormonal changes burst upon me and changed
my body almost overnight. I was a thin child at primary school but

it seemed that between the eleven-plus and the start of grammar school I swelled.

Around the age of about 15 I started reading my parents' Sunday paper. This was the sixties; 'slimming' was in. Every week there was a page on diets by Marina Andrews, whose name is graven on my heart because by that stage I was so miserable about my size that dieting beckoned with the glow of salvation and she held the key to the gates of heaven. The diets, with their promise of a slim, *acceptable* figure, were often made up of exotic ingredients which I couldn't obtain. But I could learn about calories and I did. Everyone seemed to agree that if you ate 1000 calories a day that would do the trick. I managed to eat much less than that by refusing to eat anything for supper except white fish, green beans and tomatoes: about 150 calories. I didn't eat breakfast and I picked at the school dinner. I can clearly remember the intensity of the hunger I felt during the school day and the fact that I was always cold. It wasn't just a physical coldness, though it felt like it. It was a deep, inner chill. I could not bear being different and unacceptable and my diet gave me the means to do something about it.

I don't remember when the yo-yoing started, though I do remember that I broke my diets, starving hungry and unable to resist the temptation of my mother's meat and vegetable pies (she made the most wonderful pastry). She who had tempted me with doughnuts in an attempt to expunge her guilt, now tempted me off my diets because she was worried about me. My blood sugar fell so low that I was faint, foggy in the head and in a foul mood. A meal, a *normal* meal, would make me feel as though I were emerging from unconsciousness which, in a way, I was. But then the remorse set in and it would be white fish again.

Marriage, Motherhood and Yo-yo Dieting

When I was 20 I met my husband; on my twenty-first birthday we were engaged. As a result of the draconian diets I now weighed around 13 stone. There was no shortage of encouragement to 'slim down' for the wedding, of course, and I went to my doctor, who gave me a 1000-calorie-a-day diet sheet and weighed me every week. It wasn't difficult – I had a goal, and I was very happy. I worked in Fleet Street, which had lots of little bars selling the most delicious sandwiches I have ever eaten, but they had to go (oh, turn back the clock, bid time return, just for one of those cream cheese and date sandwiches!). I used to take my lunch into work: two grapefruits, which I ate slowly at my desk, cutting them into small pieces, when everyone else had gone to the cafés and sandwich bars. By mid-afternoon, I was ravenous, but I stuck it out grimly. My future mother-in-law was a great champion of my dieting and kept me on course. I was allowed a treat every Sunday: two chocolate-covered marshmallows.

My goal was to get down to a size 16 and I had my wedding dress made that size. It hung metaphorically out of my reach while I battled down the scale of dress sizes. I cannot deny the truth: it felt wonderful to be getting thinner. I didn't want to be a fat bride and I was very aware that nobody else wanted me to be one either, apart from my future husband. He didn't care what size I was, but he encouraged me because it was what I wanted. And I got married, and I wore my dream dress and bought my going-away outfit in C & A, so proud that I didn't have to go to an outsize shop.

That was it, then. I'd reached my ideal size and weight. I didn't feel I needed to lose any more, so I stopped my diet. The GP who had overseen it had told me emphatically not to try to get below 10 stone. He was clearly a man ahead of his time, for then and now charts and BMI diagrams have dictated that I should be seven and a half to eight and a half stone. I would look horrible at that weight! As it was, I felt comely and confident in my new body.

Not long after our second wedding anniversary, I found to my huge delight that I was pregnant. I had put on weight, I knew I had, and I wasn't happy about it but I had *no idea* of the extent of the gain. At the first antenatal visit – at which time little or no weight has usually been gained – my card said that I weighed 15 stone 3 pounds. The shame of it. The sheer disbelief. How could that have happened? I had given up dieting but I hadn't been on a binge. I ate an exemplary healthy diet. Of course I had fish and chips sometimes, and cake, and the occasional chocolate bar – normal people do. I didn't count calories because normal people don't. My body had lost any sense of stability it might once have had and was now a victim of the yo-yo effect. I am as certain as anyone could be that, had I not dieted from the age of 15, I would have settled at a size 16, perhaps rising to 18 in middle age since it is entirely normal to put on a bit of weight around and after the menopause. Even though I am only 5′ 3″, I believe I was meant to be big, but not as big as I became after dieting.

There was no way I could accept the fact that I weighed over 15 stone. To put things in an historical context, this was the early seventies and obesity was far from being as prevalent as it is now. Not only were fewer people fat but those who were did not reach the high weights that are now widespread, so this should be seen through the lens of relativity. In fact, the hugely fat teacher I had at grammar school was, I now see from photographs, only about 15 stone. It's not so much that I was seeing her size with the perception of a child, though that may have played a part, but more that a 15-stone woman in those days was not that frequent a sight.

So I embarked on another diet. I learned that the baby would come to no harm; that she would receive all the nutrition she needed and would not suffer. This one was difficult; pregnancy makes you hungry. But just before delivery I weighed less than at the beginning. In fact I was told that I must eat more because I had ketones in my urine. Never before had I been told to eat more!

Our bodies behave differently at different stages and circumstances in our lives and I believe that this is largely a mysterious process. I can recall times in my adult life when clearly I was not on a diet and yet my weight remained lowish and constant. The three or so years after my first pregnancy was one such time. Having delivered my first child with all her baggage, I weighed around 12 stone. I was slightly less than that after my second daughter was born two and a half years later.

Then I began to put on weight for no discernible reason. I wanted a third child but I had reached 16 stone and I was warned against becoming pregnant at that weight. I had put on nearly five stone in three years. It sounds disingenuous to say that I don't know how it happened, but it's the truth. I enjoyed food and ate well and probably finished the leavings on the children's plates as many mothers do, and I believe now that the years of dieting destroyed my body's ability to fine tune itself and maintain a stable weight, or even to put on a little weight in response to careless eating. The much-dieted body is crying out in panic: give it a feast and it will horde as though for a siege, for it has received too many warnings that famine has arrived and conservation of fat is necessary for survival.

My desire for a baby was clearly greater than my concern about the weight and I conceived without intending to. I still feel anger and pain at the way I was treated. The first doctor I saw, for confirmation of pregnancy, said 'I hope to God you're not pregnant at that weight.' She did an examination and said I was not. She dismissed me with more harsh words, not attempting to conceal her disgust, and I felt humiliated, degraded and desperate. I knew I was pregnant and later discovered that a hormone deficiency was responsible for the absence of signs of pregnancy. This had to be treated with twice-weekly injections or I would have lost my baby son and a district nurse came to the house to administer these. It was a dreadfully painful ordeal and I don't mean physically. This woman hated fatness. She loathed and despised it and saw no reason to keep her opinion to herself. Each time she came she harassed, condemned and rebuked me for being pregnant. And she hinted darkly that a termination might be desirable.

Then there were the antenatal visits. The theme was always the same: I should not be pregnant. As if I could rewrite history. There is no doubt in my mind that had I capitulated and said yes, I'm too fat to be pregnant, let's get rid of it, I would have had no difficulty in obtaining a termination, even though it was not as easily come by then as it is now. Sometimes medical students would be invited to palpate my abdomen; this prefaced by 'If you can find the baby underneath all that blubber.' There was much snide giggling.

Why did I endure it? Because I was young, I knew nothing of assertiveness and I was vulnerable in the way that all pregnant women are vulnerable. Now, with experience and age and a history of campaigning for size acceptance and an end to prejudice, I would not let those people get away with what they did. All I can do is to urge other women who find themselves the recipients of such abuse not to endure it and to complain to the General Medical Council or the General Nursing Council. While fatness is no more tolerated now than then, there is an awareness, at least in the governing bodies of the medical profession, that bullying is unacceptable.

But I dieted, of course. I had a need to placate my abusers because I felt the safety of my baby lay in their hands. I even thought that they might not take care of his fragile intrauterine existence if I did not show that I was making amends for my sin. The pregnancy was complicated and I nearly lost him more than once. I needed their expertise and felt I had to do something in return. The memory of the shame that had rushed through me at that first ever antenatal visit, when I weighed over 15 stone, had never left me. I had kept the card in the bathroom cabinet and when I had delivered my little daughter, having lost all that weight, I believed I would never ever be as fat as that again. I looked back to my pre-wedding days when I had reached 13 stone, which had seemed mountainous. I could never have dreamed that only a few years later I'd be three stone heavier. And so, when I was due to deliver my son, I weighed less than I had at the beginning of his pregnancy.

If I close my eyes and regress I can feel again the terrible, gnawing hunger of pregnancy, a hunger I could never allow myself to satisfy. I would count the hours till lunchtime, when I permitted myself a cup of thin, low-calorie soup plus two slices of Slimcea bread: about 200 calories in all. During that last pregnancy my blood sugar, which had always been unnaturally low, was found in hospital tests to be alarmingly so. But it's true that the baby takes what he needs: my son was nearly 10 lbs.

He was born in 1978 and for the next ten years my weight continued to yo-yo. I had slimmish periods when I was around 13 stone. It is all so relative. When I first hit 13 stone I thought I first was an elephant but, having been 16 stone, 13 seemed quite desirable.

Being Fat Is Not a Sin

In 1988, working as a writer on *She* magazine, I wrote an article which they titled 'Being Fat Is Not a Sin – a Plea for an End to Prejudice'. It was the first piece to raise the issue in a mainstream magazine and it was an angry polemic about the unopposed discrimination meted out to fat people in our society. It got a huge response and I went on to write a book of the same name.[1] Because this was an issue that had not been discussed in political terms in this country, and because it is a subject on which everyone has opinions, most of them very strong, the book and I got a great deal of publicity. I took an objective stance; I spoke on behalf of all the large women and men who did not have a voice. I demanded change and equality of treatment in every context. It was not difficult; the discrimination and prejudice are so blatant. Society has been restrained in its desire to hit out at other minorities but the fat are still easy targets and have few advocates.

There was usually a personal element in these interviews, where I was asked about my feelings about my own weight. Often the assumption was made that because I had written a book calling for size acceptance, a book which said that fat people were equal to others in every way and maybe better than some at things like sensitivity and tolerance, then I must be happy being fat. I was bemused. I had never said that but I went along with it, not agreeing in so many words but claiming that the person I was had nothing to do with my size or weight and that I had achieved everything I had wanted to. That I was happy in myself, in fact. I could state with absolute truth that my husband, my children and my real friends did not care one whit whether I was fat, thin or cuboid; that, where it mattered, I was judged on many things but never on my size. What I did not say was that I disliked being so very fat. I felt that if I admitted to that the power of my message would somehow be weakened. In fact, it should have made it stronger if anything, for it is precisely because of the pain it causes that prejudice must be stamped out and I shall never cease to campaign for this. But, I found it immensely painful to talk about my size when I was a high weight. It was almost as though I thought that if I didn't talk about it people wouldn't notice it. As if! But I avoided saying anything that might draw attention to it and perhaps provoke questions that I would not be comfortable answering. The fact is though that if you are a big woman and you write a polemical, angry book saying that society should accept fat people as they are then it is assumed that you yourself are happy with your size. So I kept quiet.

Although I was very large I had always been very fit. Then I began to feel weak and exhausted. We live at the top of a steep hill and I had always walked up it fast as a form of daily exercise, but it became insurmountable. In the space of about a year, I went from having normal fitness and mobility to hardly being able to drag myself 50 yards along a flat stretch. In 1992, I was diagnosed with ME and for about a year I was virtually bedridden.

My body, which thanks to the years of yo-yo dieting was forever looking for a chance to increase itself – give it an inch and it would put on six! – immediately responded to the enforced immobility and in five years I put on three stone. And in doing so I crossed a barrier in my own mind that I hadn't even known was there. I think every woman has this barrier: it's the weight above which it is definitely unacceptable to be. Not unacceptable to society – though it may be that, too – but something much more subjective. For Rosemary Conley it was when she hit 10 st 3 lbs at her fattest. Now I would feel a bit waiflike at 10 st 3 lbs, which, given that we are about the same height, shows just *how* personal and subjective this whole self-image thing is.

For me, this concept was something to do with hating being fat while still managing to take my place in the world and believing I should be acceptable and accepted there. That sounds like a contradiction and it may be, but it is the only way I can describe it.

Around this time, I wrote a letter to a much-loved friend. This friend, also an author, had written something I considered fattist and offensive. Though it was not about me, I took it personally, thinking huh, so that's how she sees me, some friend. She accepted my criticism of the way she had expressed herself in her book, but she threw me a tough question. 'How can you expect me to accept your size when you don't accept it yourself?' she wrote back. It was a bit of a blinding flash: an illumination of the perversity of what I was demanding of the world at large. Of course size acceptance should be a given. But she was right: was it logical or even fair to ask people to like my body when I didn't like it myself? Though I didn't know it at the time, her question – a question that I felt deserved an answer – had sown the seed for change in me.

The Political and the Personal: Facing a Decision

I was 19$^1/_2$ stone and I felt utterly gross. I could look at other women of that weight – and much heavier – and find them beautiful and graceful, but I felt that I was unacceptable to myself. Although prior to that my confidence had only been superficial, it had got me by. Now that had deserted me. I couldn't even undress in front of my husband. All these years I had been reading letters in women's magazines saying just that – usually from women who were a size 18. I thought they were ridiculous. How could you hate your own body that much, I had asked rhetorically, but now it was happening to me. I went from just disliking my photograph being taken to feeling real pain and panic if it happened and I couldn't avoid it without making a scene. I didn't like being touched and I would dress and undress without looking at any part of my body. If I had died at that time, those were the images I could not have borne to leave to posterity.

Having ME certainly exacerbated all this. Not only did it cause further weight gain, but the immobility turned me, in my own mind, into a symbol of how we as fat people are perceived by society at large. When I was quick and agile it was easy to refute the stereotype of slow, lazy, clumsy, waddling, etc, but that was exactly what ME forced upon me. A doctor, sent to evaluate me for a car mobility badge, reported me as having the 'typical rolling gait of the very obese'. It painted such a hideous picture that I could not get his words out of my mind and saw myself, on the world's stage, shuffling and rolling from side to side with wobbling acres of flesh.

Unknown to anyone, even my husband, I had been doing a little research into weight-loss methods. I was worried about the idea of going on a diet, for a multitude of reasons. I'd done it before, hadn't I? And it had never worked. I'd lost weight certainly but gained it back with interest. Such a typical scenario and one I've had described to me by so many women over the years since my first book was published. I knew one thing for certain: if I was to embark on any weight-loss programme it must be for the last time. I could not endure going through all the loss and regain again. I was 51; if I didn't lose weight now, I thought, I never would. I'd go into old age (presuming I had an old age to go into) as a very large woman and I simply did not want to be a very large woman any more. Equally, for psychological and health reasons, I didn't want to be a failed dieter yet again.

I was in a quandary. The idea of weight loss meant stepping outside at least one of my comfort zones: the one that spoke the received wisdom that diets don't work, that it is safer to remain a stable, high weight than to lose and regain and that the most important thing was to eat a thoroughly healthy diet.

Years before, I had met Jill Welbourne, who was then running a clinic for eating disorders. When I started writing about weight issues, she was my mentor and expert. She had counselled me about my own eating. 'Don't diet,' she said, 'just promise yourself that you will only put into your mouth foods that are good for your body.' I had thought it excellent advice and had followed it. But healthy eating does not make you lose weight, nor does it keep your weight stable if you eat too much good food and don't exercise enough.

I loved my breakfast the most: a big bowl of homemade muesli with an abundance of nuts, seeds and all kinds of dried fruit, eaten with natural yogurt. I dreaded having to give that up. I feared any kind of deprivation. One very powerful thread running through my life has been fear of starvation. Not literally, but anyone who has dieted at a young age when mind and body are still forming – dieted to the extent that most of the day is spent physically hungry – will have acquired this fear, consciously or not. It's an atavistic alarm bell that we should not need in this time of plenty but which can be set, as mine was, by the very real famines to which I subjected myself as a young teenager. With me it is exacerbated by my abnormally low blood sugar, which makes me feel faint and dizzy and has on one occasion led to coma. When I feel it falling, like a fast lift, I get a bit panicky.

Apart from all that – and all that was rather a lot in itself – there were the beliefs I had acquired during my years of writing about size acceptance. I had met so many outstanding people in the movement and I had become even more convinced of the rightness of our stance. Not only for political reasons: I had read a great deal of scientific research that claimed that the stated health risks of being overweight were at best exaggerated, at worst simply not true. This was a dastardly ploy by the fat-hating medical profession to rid the world of the dreaded obese. Then there was the literature on the dangers of dieting – very real, physical dangers, some life-threatening – and all the empirical evidence that 95 per cent of weight lost is regained. What chance had I? Why should I be any different?

I turned that figure on its head. If 95 per cent of weight was regained, then 5 per cent was not. Why should I *not* be in that 5 per cent?

But the idea of weight loss felt so alien. I had said so many times in interviews that I would never diet again and though I had misled people about being happy with my weight, I was reconciled to accepting that I would be this way for the rest of my life. And I despised the whole diet culture: the narcissistic obsession with size and shape; the assertions that no one could be successful, healthy, sexy, attractive or even likeable if they were overweight; the arrogance of the belief that only one kind of body was acceptable. I didn't have to go along with that, though, and I never will. After all, these people are talking about thinness as the only desirable goal and I don't want to be thin. I would remain anarchic by simply wanting to be less fat, though that put me between the devil of the thin-worshipping, finger-wagging mainstream society and the deep blue sea of the size-acceptance movement, emphasis on *acceptance*.

During the time I was reflecting on these things, I was working on *Sizeable Reflections*,[2] a book celebrating the lives and achievements of a couple of dozen fabulous big women. Each of them was contributing an original essay to the anthology and I realised, reading them, that my ambivalence was not so unusual. While many of the contributors expressed a fierce pride in their size, others touched on the pain of being fat. But none had allowed it to inhibit the course of their lives, and triumph over considerable adversity was the keynote of several of the essays. Together they made a joyful and moving collection. The courage and the feistiness of the women were inspiring; by the time the book was completed I counted them all as friends.

The title of my essay, 'The Devil and the Deep Blue Sea', indicated my ambivalence. It began: 'I am afraid of being thin', and it went on to explore the difficulties of being very fat and yet not wanting to be the size prescribed by the society we live in. I also wrote about my fear of being rejected should I ever admit to my desire to be thinner.

Through my work I came to realise that there are many shades of grey between the black and white certainties of fat hatred and fat pride. What is often not recognised is that some of us – and I know now that I am one – would like to he less fat than we are. Once I identified my feelings about my size I did not dare share them … I thought that if I confessed to my colleagues in the size-acceptance movement that I was not entirely comfortable with my bulk, then they might ostracise me.

In fact, understanding my true position has been a source of enormous liberation. I have broken the bonds of two different but equally confining ideals.

And so the secret I had kept even from myself was well and truly out. I could not go on accepting my size. There was another matter, too. I had read and written countless times about the facts and myths about health and weight as far as they can be disentangled. There is so much evidence that fatness is not the health hazard it is trumped up to be. But I have never ever been able to feel that in my very large body I was as safe as someone who weighed several stone less than me. I did not feel that conviction that I was at no more risk of diabetes, cancer or heart disease than the 10-stone woman. The studies I had read which showed that the longest life was enjoyed by those who were about 30 per cent overweight did not bring comfort to me for I was about 100 per cent over, according to those damn charts on which such studies are based.

Although I knew how to lose weight I was also aware of the importance of support. Losing weight alone leaves you open to boredom, despair and self-sabotage. Unfortunately, the NHS, while preaching in best nanny-state fashion to those of us who weigh more than we should, provides little or nothing in the way of support for those who do want to do something about it. I'd been to Weight Watchers twice in my previous dieting life and hadn't liked it. I lasted for only one meeting.

Extract from diary, September 1982

Tried a Weight Watchers class. I hated the emphasis on What Is Important. The class lecturer said that when I had lost weight I would really take an interest in looking good, in going to the hairdresser, etc. I replied that I never went to the hairdresser because my husband had always cut my hair. 'Ah, but that will change,' she said knowingly.

*How patronising can you get! And the rebel in me cannot cope with
'On week two you will be allowed rice with your vegetables...' or
'When you reach goal weight you can have your favourite meal.'
Thanks very much. I'm actually not four years old. The worst thing,
though, was when she gave me my goal weight of eight stone four. I
said very politely that I did not want to go as low as that and would
rather set it at about eleven stone. 'You'll have to bring a letter from
your doctor if you want to do that', the old bat said. So I shan't be
going again. How do these women stand being spoken to like
imbeciles/children/subhuman citizens? It seems that getting fat denies
you the right to be treated with normal intelligence or courtesy.*

But I'd read a lot of good things about Slimming World, including
the fact that its members claimed never to be hungry. Could I do it,
I wondered? In fact, I wondered for about two years. I had written
a round condemnation of the exploitative diet industry and I
disliked the idea of a slimming club. I'm not a group person at the
best of times and anyway how could I compromise my principles?

In the end self-preservation won over principles, though in the
eyes of some activists I compromised my integrity as a campaigner
by deciding to lose weight. I maintain that the ideal of a just world
and the desire to be thinner are not mutually exclusive themes.

I did my research and decided to give Slimming World a go.

The Last-chance Diet

At the beginning of November 1998, I went with my family for
the Centre Parcs weekend described in Chapter Two. I ate well,
mentally saying farewell to my favourite things, including the
chestnut pie I made and took with us. We returned from Centre
Parcs on Monday and on Tuesday at midday I turned up for my
local Slimming World class, using a pseudonym. I didn't want
anyone to know that I was the author of *The Forbidden Body*.

Extract from diary, 10 November 1998
*Like a lamb to the slaughter I go to Slimming World. First thing I
notice is that nobody else is fat! Even among my 'peers' I feel different.
One other new member, a prissy woman in her sixties, size 10–12. Has
joined in order to lose half a stone. I hate her on sight. Class consultant*

very nice. After weighing we have 'Image Therapy' sitting in a circle. I sit next to a comfortable, middle-aged woman who has to lose weight for a back operation. She gives me her life history and a recipe: Line a flan dish bottom and sides with corned beef, beat six eggs and add them, top with mashed potato and bake in the oven. She points out that corned beef and eggs are 'free foods', meaning you can eat them without restriction. Surely not? Rose, the consultant, reads a piece about a day in the life of a dieter who picked her way though 50 'sins' (the 'plan' allows 10 a day) and wondered why she hadn't lost weight. Then everyone's weight loss is read out and we applaud each one. Very cosy. I feel out of place.

After that class Rose explained the Slimming World system to me with its combination of free foods, healthy extras and sins. It meant a lot of looking up food values in the book but I found I soon got to know them by heart. It's a combination of counting the healthy extras and 'sins' and not counting the free food. I discovered I liked this, the mix of control and freewheeling. I liked the idea that the eating plan was formulated to avoid feelings of deprivation.

Extract from diary – Class 2, 17 November 1998

Lining up for the weigh-in I feel such a failure. My skirt is tight and I know I haven't lost any weight. Then I get on the scales, not looking. Rose tells me to get off and then on again. She stares hard then writes something down, then looks at me. 'You've lost ten pounds!' I feel faint – hunger? – and embarrassed. During Image Therapy the class is told. But I know it won't stay off. I've lost it too fast. I wanted to lose one pound a week. There is a raffle and I win the prize – a grapefruit. The only raffle I've ever won and I get a grapefruit! The language used here is that of dieters everywhere: being good, sinning, cheating. I've always hated it, always felt women shouldn't have to use the language of wrongdoing where weight loss is concerned, that they only do so because they are reflecting social prejudice and condemnation. Judged and found wanting. But I do want to lose weight. Decide I can only benefit from all this by playing the game.

At Slimming World you are encouraged to set yourself a series of goal weights so that your achievement is measured in steps rather than in one great leap, which could take months or even years. When you have six or seven stone to lose that ultimate target weight can seem depressingly unrealistic not to mention unattainable. My first goal was to lose three stone, even that seemed ambitious for it meant that if I did it I would be 16+ stone – a weight I had not been for many years.

Extract from diary, 22 March 1999

Have lost 1 stone 13lbs. This crazy diet works, in spite of eating unlimited macaroni cheese! Woman being weighed today looked completely normal weight. Bah humbug! Am aware of the importance of exercise but it's not easy with ME. *Nevertheless have started walking a bit every day. It wouldn't be so bad but for the steep hills round here.*

The 'eating plan' worked because the psychology of dieting and dieters has been studied and identified by Slimming World. Most 'eating plans' today are conscious of the 'diets don't work' theory that sprang up in the eighties and of the uselessness of having 'forbidden foods'. Slimming World's stroke of genius is its concept of 'free foods'. It's no good telling people that they can have as much salad (with non-fat dressing) as they want or that they can eat broccoli until it's coming out of their ears. There are few people who love salad or broccoli to that extent and the fact is that vegetables are not, on the whole, satisfying.

The Slimming World free foods seem, at first glance, quite outrageous! There is no restriction on eggs, meat, fish, vegetables, fruit, some cheeses and a whole range of branded products. If you want to eat a whole chicken at a sitting, you can. If you want to guzzle two tins of macaroni cheese (the thing I developed a passion for at the beginning) you can.

I was deeply sceptical. It would never have occurred to me before to eat tinned macaroni cheese because it was high in fat. However, it beckoned once I started the diet. Pasta in cheese sauce, very satisfying. I'd lived most of my life in fear of 'forbidden foods' and the notion that some of these were now unrestricted was like opening the door for a caged lion. I took it all quite literally, even thought I'd show them that their 'plan' didn't work. But I lost weight because the free foods were a sort of dietary 'loss leader'. If you could have them in quantity, you actually didn't eat them in quantity but you were freed from the fear of hunger. And – most importantly – they allowed for comfort eating. Everyone comfort eats – or drinks – sometimes. The point about most diets is that you can't do it. If I wanted to comfort eat I would choose a small tin of macaroni cheese. I still lost weight because without really trying I was self-regulating my intake. And after a while the macaroni cheese palled. The reason I had fallen for such a processed and not very healthy food was that this was the kind of food I had either been denying myself or eating guiltily all my life. To be able to eat it freely was liberation indeed.

I lost weight very slowly. In two and a half years I have lost six and a half stone. That's less than one pound a week and would not be fast enough for many people, but I am doing this for life and I want to maximise my chances of keeping it off. Fast weight loss never lasts. I lost the first stone in only a month. The second took three and a half months; the third (my first goal) another three. Three stone in seven and a half months. The fourth stone took another three and a half months; the fifth, four months; and the sixth stone took an arduous and often despairing ten months. The last half stone took a few more, and I have decided to maintain 13 stone.

Extract from diary, 8 June 1999

Have struggled for many weeks now. Weight plateaued and even went up a couple of times. But now I've lost 4 lbs in a fortnight and am at last below 17 stone – first time in about 12 years. Wonderful feeling.

As your weight falls so does the number of calories at which your body will burn its fat stores. This is a very tough fact of dieting life; you do your body a favour and it just says okay, I need even less now. During the two years I hit a number of depressing plateaus on which I stuck for weeks. The free food principle no longer worked for me, though I still appreciate it and it has been my salvation. But I have passions – all for 'good' foods – but all foods contain calories. I live near an apple farm, I love apples, but I don't think when Slimming World dreamed up the free food idea it meant eating eight apples a day. It's tough, knowing I could put the weight back on by overdoing such things as apples, beetroot and dried apricots and prunes. It makes me angry, too, when I think of the commonly held stereotype of fat people's eating; the firmly held belief that to get fat we must be consuming cream cakes, chocolate and high-fat junk food like burgers and chips. I'm here to tell you that in order to keep my weight down I have to watch my consumption of fruit and veg!

Extract from diary, 14 September 1999

Feeling despondent and stuck. Goal of 15 stone by Christmas not attainable as am 16 stone now. Weight loss has slowed down and calorie intake dropped. Now feels like hard work without reward. So need to remind myself that I have lost 3¹/₂ stone in 10 months and goal was 4 stone in a year. Should lose 7 lbs by Christmas, which would be 4 stone in just over a year. That would be good. Although weight loss seems slow, looking back my record shows that I have lost 11 lbs in three months, just under 1 lb a week, which isn't bad. The previous three months show a 1-stone loss, slightly faster (and on more calories). So I must just keep going. However slow, it will go and this time next year I could be 13–14 stone – brilliant! Need to keep the exercise up too. Every day a 35-minute walk which seems uphill all the way there and most of the way back. Not my favourite part of the day.

Losing weight, even on a diet that does not entail severe calorie depletion, is very, very hard. It is about denial and deprivation because it has to be. Holidays, special occasions and meals out are very difficult. At Christmas I was so frightened of putting on weight I just ate turkey, sprouts and carrots with a little gravy. No stuffing, Christmas pudding or cake or mince pies. I lost my usual pound over the two-week period. Then Easter came and that was much more difficult. I wasn't too bothered about the chocolate but warm, spicy, fruity hot cross buns – that was another matter! On Good Friday in our house we tend to eat them for breakfast, elevenses and tea. So I decided to have a binge. I allowed myself 15 hot cross buns that day – and nothing else. They were half fat and the day's supply came to about 3,000 calories.

I thought I'd be in raptures but I discovered something I'd never encountered in myself before. I was much happier when I was on my diet, however difficult I was finding it. I've never been a control freak but now I realised that the idea of controlling my food was important.

Extract from diary, Good Friday, 2000

Decided to appease cravings by having an entire day of hot cross buns and no other food. Surprised by anxiety – felt out of control when I started my breakfast buns. Wondered if I even wanted to go through with it. Realised the comfort and safety of sticking to the diet. This feels like the slippery slope to disaster. Felt I'd put on pounds after four hot cross buns!

There were times when I simply lost it.

Extract from diary, 18 April 2000

Bad food day – needs analysing. I've been so cold and tired, and hungry in a way that I haven't been on the diet till now – feeling of not being satisfied. Could be partly due to very thin bread for breakfast. Trying to fill up with apples but eating too many. Teatime was the lowest point of the day. Ate sugar-free jelly and a banana. Not satisfied. Feeling hunger of all kinds. Peanut butter sandwich led to peanut butter binge which I could have controlled but went ahead. Huge regret but maybe necessary. Watch out for winter blues and tiredness. Eat free food if feel like that again.

It was true – the peanut butter feast was necessary. I never needed to do it again. And I realised that any diet that says you shouldn't eat unless you are really hungry doesn't understand human emotions and our complex relationship with food. If I had eaten satisfying 'free food' earlier in the day, the teatime binge wouldn't have happened. I was learning all the time.

Extract from diary, 20 August 2000

Have experienced surges of urges this last couple of days. Had to eat Parmesan while making pesto. Ate too much pasta and sauce at supper, big plateful, didn't need it. But routine is upset and stress predominates. What is important is to remember that I have eaten in a way that has lost me over five stone so it can be done. Cravings to eat can be satisfied with free food and fruit and jelly have been excellent standbys. The urge to eat too much can be controlled by not eating a lot – the appetite grows by what it feeds on! If I 'break' the diet I only feel bad. Nothing was gained by eating 3 oz Parmesan – except extra weight. One ounce would have been sufficient. Threw some pasta away – hard to be convinced that it's better in the bin (waste!) than in my stomach, but it is. Keeping on the plan steadily actually removes addictive tendencies, but it's important not to be totally deprived of treats all the time because that just leads to break-out bingeing. Hard sometimes to get the balance right.

I was very secretive about my weight loss. I only told my family and a few very close friends what I was doing. I don't like being the centre of attention in any event and I could not bear the scrutiny or the remarks that might come my way. There is a certain amount of ambivalence about losing weight and I experienced both extremes of emotion. I felt very fiercely that I didn't want to be praised for any loss I might achieve because I was hypersensitive to the implicit criticism of the person I was before that loss. I didn't want to tell people because I thought they would watch me and pass positive comments which would make me want to say 'So what was wrong with me when I was fatter?' I felt excruciatingly aware of the fact that people, on the whole, do think you're somehow a better person when you lose weight. I felt a great need to protect the wounded fat person that I was, even if that person was about to become thinner.

But I was hoist by my own petard! When I'd lost two stone, having been truculently opposed to anyone commenting on it, I had to face the fact that no one *was* going to comment because no one had noticed! This was because the harsh fact is that if you are very large, over 19 stone in my case, you do not look so very different at 17 stone! Two stones' worth of hard work and nobody notices! I couldn't even tell! I felt just the same, my clothes, always loose and concealing, felt the same. One day I was talking to one of the friends I had confided in. 'I know what I keep meaning to ask you,' she said. 'Did you ever go to Slimming World or did you change your mind?' Collapse of stout party! As she is a very close friend we were able to laugh and agree that at my size, two stone was a mere drop in the ocean of abundant flesh.

I asked my husband if he could tell I'd lost two stone. He couldn't but I didn't blame him for that. He has never cared about my size, doesn't see me as a fat or even less fat woman. He just sees me as me, so his not noticing was simply indicative of that.

When I'd lost three stone and still no one remarked on it, I was miffed. I was in a perverse state of mind because for the reason given above I didn't want to be complimented, but I did want people to notice. I planned that if anyone did say anything, I would act surprised. 'Lost weight?' I'd say. 'Oh, I don't think so. It must be this dress.' But the fact was that I can't deny that I was now feeling so much better about myself. Three stone of the hated fat had gone and I wanted to share my pleasure – but on my terms! My poor friends were damned if they did comment and damned if they didn't. But they were more damned if they didn't.

A couple of the people in the know suggested that perhaps the weight loss *had* been noticed but that friends were refraining from making remarks for the very reason I had wanted them not to do so. What a number of people had said was how well I was looking. As I had all but recovered from ME (following the discovery of a long-standing gas leak in the house, which gives food for thought on that particular illness), I had assumed that the remarks were to do with that. But my daughters insisted that 'You look so well' was a euphemism for 'You've lost weight'. I think they were right.

Then people did start to remark on the weight loss, though by this time I'd lost five stone and they could hardly have failed to notice. My pride would not let me admit that I had done it deliberately and intentionally; it felt far too personal, an admission that I hadn't liked myself before. I also felt extremely strongly that I did not want people to think that my weight loss was a tacit acceptance of the social mandate that women should not be fat. My beliefs about people's right to be the size they are is stronger than ever, if anything. On the other hand, there was no getting away from the fact that I was absolutely ecstatic that I'd lost so much and did enjoy people's compliments. There is no doubt – and this is a sad fact – that I like myself better now. I tried to learn to love my body when I was very fat but I just couldn't manage it.

My efforts to stay cool, to evince surprise when people commented, led me one day when someone accosted me in the street and shrieked about how much weight I'd lost, to say 'Have I?' in very surprised tones. 'Oh, dear,' she said. 'You're not ill or anything, are you?' I'm afraid I may have left the poor woman under the impression that I had some awful disease and that she'd put her foot in it. I was not being deliberately provocative when I feigned surprise or ignorance or casual disregard. It was all too close to me at the time.

Losing weight has, for me, been a quiet revolution. I have much more confidence, more mobility, more agility and I can – almost – bear to look in a mirror. I feel physically and psychologically better and no amount of political correctness can deny that. The fact is, though, that in some ways nothing has changed. I am still a large woman, still someone whom doctors will harass and many will despise. I haven't stepped out of the arena of size-acceptance politics. I am just a medium-fat woman instead of a supersized one. I think, medically, I am still what they so charmingly term 'grossly obese'. I am roughly the weight I was when I *began* my wedding diet in 1968, when I perceived myself as pretty monstrous and couldn't face the idea of walking up the aisle at that size.

I am happy with my weight. (How many women of 13 stone would say that, I wonder?) I am under no illusions as to how hard maintenance is going to be. Every day I am aware that my body is fighting to put the weight back on again. I can almost feel it physically. At the moment I seem to be running just to stand still.

Extract from diary, 24 October 2000

The wedding party was difficult – full of tempting, comforting, satisfying foods like quiche and sausage rolls. The food scared me so I ate nothing, not even a piece of the celebration cake. Maybe this iron will to refuse to weaken at all *times could be the downfall as it all went horribly wrong on Sunday morning. I had to get up early to put the party food away and the will power broke. I started eating against my will, couldn't stop. The fact that it was only four small sausage rolls is immaterial, it was the feeling of being controlled by the* 'autre' *as in Rimbaud's* 'Je et un autre.' *Any event which takes me outside the framework of my acquired 'good' eating habits seems to threaten the whole structure.*

I am still not interested in most discussion about weight because the larger part of it is about bemoaning the state of being a size 12 when you want to be a 10 or preferably an 8; it is small talk about the high-protein diet and doesn't Jennifer Aniston look great or about the fact that you ate too much chocolate at Christmas and put on 3 lbs. That *is* boring. I have always said that there are two kinds of weight problem: the one I have where your body overflows the medical and social boundaries set for its acceptability – anything above 12 stone, to give a rough figure – and the one where you don't cross these boundaries but want to be thin because our mindless social aesthetic is that thin is not only best, it is the only acceptable way to be.

I can't be sure about my future. I know this has to be the last time I lose weight. I know I can never come off the diet, never again eat normally. I'm aware of the importance of staying focused, of keeping my eye on this particular ball, particularly now I'm maintaining a stable weight. It's about habit and routine, about keeping a certain mindset and remaining in a constant state of alertness. I intend to carry on at Slimming World because it means that once a week I have that sharp focus. I never did become an enthusiastic class member. This was not the fault of the consultant nor the method, simply a reflection of the fact that I am a loner rather than a group animal. I noticed that some people slipped into class, got weighed then left. I started doing this myself, knowing that if I wanted the group support I could stay any time. I do like the camaraderie that exists between members, the way you know that everyone is rooting for you. Sometimes, if things seem difficult, I stay to class and it always helps. As in most situations, much can be learned from the experiences of other travellers in the same boat. Often I come away with a host of practical suggestions and excellent recipes, though I never have made the corned beef flan.

I have learned the value of support, though, which I got and still get from Rose, the consultant. It has convinced me that weight loss without support is such a lonely and difficult furrow to plough that it is virtually impossible.

If I dare hope it is because all the other diets had endings: they stopped when I reached my goal. This has to be for life.

Extract from diary, 30 January 2001

It's so important to keep everything in mind at this point. I can see how easy it would be to let go – to stop counting, to relax the discipline, to have two date and apricot rolls because I like them so much. The weight could so easily pile back on. So remember: the SW plan works; calorie counting works; eating too little doesn't work but eating plenty of the right food does. No need to go hungry. But don't get slack. Don't have meals out without counting, sacrifice where possible, and compensate. Don't eat something just because others are – or not often. Keep the diet in focus. Don't let it slip or the edges blur.

One thing I have to live with is that although I have lost six and a half stone it makes no difference to society's perception of me. I am still a fat woman, still a moral transgressor. The prejudice will remain. So the gains have to be big enough and important enough to make weight loss an imperative for reasons other than social acceptability.

Yes, it's tough. But it's my choice. It may not be yours but I hope the rest of this book will help you decide what you want to do. If you have a great deal of weight to lose then, like me, after two years of long-haul dieting, you'll still be fat and will have to decide whether you want to go on. Don't ever be fooled by 'experts' who tell you that all you have to do is change your lifestyle, as though that were some painless magic formula. You *will* have to change it: you'll have to be punctilious about taking exercise even if you don't want to and you'll have to stick to a diet.

Personally, I think it's worth it. For me the rewards are much greater than the drawbacks, however much I might moan about them.

Maintenance

If I were to tell you what I want, what I really, really want, I suppose I would say I'd like to weigh 10 stone-ish. That would be perfection. But in order to do this I would have to cut down my calorie intake, increase my exercise and generally start punishing myself.

I'm not prepared to do that. I am happy with my body and that is *all* that matters. What a lifetime of being fat has taught me is that not only is perfection unattainable, but the search for it is destructive. If perfection is the goal, that goal is never reached. It is strange to think that for two of the women featured in this book, Esther Rantzen and Rosemary Conley, 10 stone-ish was the weight they were unhappy with. I would feel very dainty at that weight but know I could not reach it. But there's a great deal to be said for the 'good enough' principle: like Winnicott's concept of the 'good enough mother' (another area of women's lives where we want to be perfect). It removes discontented strivings for something that does not exist.

I am still too fat by the yardstick (or tape measure or set of scales!) of the medical profession and society in general, but who cares? Not me, not my family nor my friends, so no one else matters. Though I used to *believe* that to be true when I was nearly 20 stone, I could not turn that intellectual conviction into everyday living. But I am now a large woman who is content to remain large. In this respect I feel I have become a fuller, more honest part of the size-acceptance movement; I can at last say I'm happy to be the way I am.

I am still on a diet: that can never change if I want to maintain this weight. I still keep a food diary which I find helpful, not a chore. The feelings of deprivation have lessened considerably because my restricted eating has become a familiar pattern. It helps to remember that human beings are both creatures of habit and infinitely adaptable. I have adapted to my new eating habits and they seem – almost – normal. After all, I have been eating this way for nearly three years now. I no longer find it difficult when other people eat 'fattening' foods in front of me, though if I am hungry, smells can be a problem! As can walking through the supermarket (never go to the shops on an empty stomach!)

The way I eat on 'maintenance' is slightly different from the weight-loss part of the diet. My basic eating plan is still the same. I still rob Peter to pay Paul: if I have a meal out I will cut back the next day. I don't feel that eating out is the problem it was: previously a couple of meals out during a week meant that there was no weight loss that week. Now that I am not trying to lose weight I can take in those meals. I don't necessarily mean in restaurants, but supper with friends. Meals out have become a great treat. When I was very large I never enjoyed them because I always felt I 'shouldn't' be having them. Now, because they are special, they are not part of my diet. In a restaurant I will choose a lower-calorie option but not necessarily something as spartan as grilled fish and salad. The other night I opted for spaghetti bolognese – what I really wanted was the three cheese and broccoli bake! – but maintaining weight loss and having what you want aren't really compatible.

This may still sound like deprivation and to some extent it has to be. I know I can never eat normally and I can't emphasise that enough. If I did – if I ever do – I would just become part of the 95 per cent recidivism statistic. But I enjoy my food more now simply because it *is* restricted. One particular delight is that I have started to eat butter again. I banished this from my diet around the age of 15 when I started on the treadmill of loss and regain. I thought that butter was a Very Bad Fattening Food. As I dislike all spreads, I have always eaten my toast dry. I never minded: it became a habit. But now, perhaps once a week, I have bread and butter. Food of the gods!

A typical day's eating on maintenance
Breakfast: Two pieces of wholemeal toast and low-calorie jam (no butter or spread). *About 250 calories*

Mid-morning: Apple or dried fruit. *About 100 calories*

Lunch: Vegetable soup (home-made, puréed vegetables with stock), roll, salad with olive oil dressing. *About 500 calories*

Mid-afternoon: Apple or dried fruit. *About 100 calories*

Tea: Banana or carton of natural fromage frais. *About 100 calories*

Supper: Salmon fillet, broccoli, carrots, beetroot. Apple. *About 500 calories*

Drinks: No-calorie herb tea, Diet Coke or mineral water. A small glass of fruit juice with breakfast at weekends.

This particular day comes to 1550 calories and that is on the generous side because of the olive oil in the salad. I try to average about 1500 calories a day; some days it is considerably less because I'm allowing for meals out on other days. The calorie allowances given above are over estimated; overweight people are always accused of underestimating their calorie intake, which may nor may not be true, but I find it pays to err on the right side. It has to be a pretty large apple to come to 100 calories, for example. And supermarket salmon fillets are around 250 calories so I've vastly overestimated the calorie values of the vegetables.

Like anyone who has ever been substantially overweight, I am aware that food has had an important and complex role in my life. Once food inserts itself into your emotional template, once it establishes its place as a powerful, addictive force that is very much more than just fuel for the body, I think you have to treat it with respect. There *is* a parallel with other addictions. One of the criticisms of dieting is that it makes you preoccupied with food all the time. All I can say is that you're not half as preoccupied as when food is ruling you instead of the other way round. When I was very fat I spent as much, if not more, time obsessing over my weight, what I was eating, what I should or shouldn't be eating, how I looked, how bad I felt, what people were thinking, how I wished I could be like X who only weighed 13 stone so what had she got to worry about? . . . etc, etc . . . All that thinking was entirely negative and destructive and it had no direction. Yes, I do like being in control of my weight but I see nothing wrong in that. I believe that what I am doing now, on maintenance, is what a vast number of 'normal' weight women do all the time. It's just that we don't notice them doing it because they don't get fat. Their weight fluctuates, maybe by a stone or more, but they cut back before it escalates to true fatness.

Where eating is concerned lifestyle factors always count. For me the difficulty is being at home all day, alone, often working on something very tedious or very stressful. There's no one to break the monotony or to chat things over with. I have always eaten in times of stress and this is what I have to watch out for. Again it's to do with habits and patterns; if you can identify them, you can deal with them. The brain gives you cues and associations: I cannot separate letter writing (by hand) from eating apples. I write letters at the dining-room table; there is always a big bowl of apples on that table so a long session could result in the consumption of a lot of apples. Pen in one hand, apple in the other. Just a habit, not a very terrible one but it needs watching. When you've lost weight, apples can make you gain a lot!

I still growl when I hear 'healthy eating' used as a euphemism for losing weight. My big food battles are still with dried fruit, wholemeal bread loaded with seeds and wholefood peanut butter (made from crushed peanuts, nothing added). The calories in that lot are enormous! I do eat dried fruit every day but I weigh it. One thing that has lightened my life considerably is a scale (made by Soehnle) which not only weighs food but gives you its calorie value at the same time. It is salutary to see that the small pile of dried apricots I fancy has about 200 calories when I would have guessed at around 50! No, it's not sad, it's extremely useful. Sorry, but calories *do* count.

But it isn't *all* about restriction. What I have learned is that the dieted, deprived body will give you a hard time unless you accede to its desires at times. You do need to listen to your body. Sometimes mine tells me that one ounce of dried fruit isn't enough. It says I need four or five ounces. It won't let me get on with anything, I prowl and keep going back to the cupboard... This is a binge waiting in the wings. So I pre-empt it. I eat four ounces or whatever. My body says, no – give me more. I say just wait ten minutes or so and then we'll see. After ten minutes I usually feel pretty sick (dried fruit is very rich and sweet). The longing for it then goes away for days: I suspect one day it will disappear altogether. It's a trigger food for me but not one of the dangerous ones like chocolate.

But even dangerous foods need to be accommodated. I do love chocolate. I don't eat it because of the longing it sets up. But every six months or so I feel a desperate need for it – a lot of it. So I'll buy a large bar and eat it. This has a double effect: I usually don't want anything else to eat for hours and hours. And I don't want chocolate again for months. (Actually the last time I did this was ten months ago but I don't feel a longing at the moment. Maybe it's gone.)

They – the 'experts' – tell to you to have a little of what you fancy. If that works for you, great. It works for me with the dried fruit, on the whole. But when I need my four ounces, I need it. And when I need my big bar of chocolate, a couple of squares won't do. The thing is that eating four ounces of dried fruit every couple of months and a large bar of Dairy Milk every six months to a year is *not* going to make you put on weight. Satisfying the craving does mean that you don't eat again for a long time so your calorie allowance doesn't go miles into the red. It's a safety measure: at the back of your mind you know that if and when you need it, you can have it.

Fat people, who give in to cravings, are pilloried – but then fat people are pilloried for eating anything at all. Most women of all weights have food cravings, often hormonally linked, and chocolate is one of them. I remember my daughter and her friends looking for a late-night garage once because the chocolate craving had hit them and the shops were shut. They returned armed with their booty – several bars of chocolate each. Because they are slim, people found this amusing. Same deed, different perceptions.

I am always conscious of my diet-impaired metabolism and my body's efficient 'housekeeping' – its desperate attempts to replace its depleted fat stores. I have just returned from a week's holiday in Venice. As we went with another couple it was an interesting way to experiment. Angela and I ate exactly the same except that she had ice creams and alcohol every day whereas I did not. I drank mineral water or Diet Coke. We took exactly the same exercise, walking round Venice and getting healthily exhausted.

I am heavier and younger than Angela, which means that my metabolic rate should be higher – more efficient – than hers. This, combined with the fact that I took in fewer calories, should have been reflected in our respective weight gains. She put on three pounds, I gained six.

I've stopped panicking about these things. I know they are going to happen, that when I deviate from the diet my body is going to have a field day storing up the harvest. But I also know that when I return to the diet I will get back to my working weight of 13 stone. Two weeks after our return the 6 lbs had gone again. A fair amount of it would have been water, retained because of the extra carbohydrates I consumed in the form of pasta. In Italy, a bowl of pasta is cheap and bread is free; a meal of meat or fish with vegetables is much more expensive.

I am interested in people's reactions to my six and a half stone loss. There is absolutely no doubt now that it is noticeable. Some people still have not remarked on it but I no longer speculate on why that might be. I am sure my daughter is right and that comments on how well I am looking can be translated into 'because you've lost so much weight'! Since reaching 13 stone, several people, independently of each other, have expressed an opinion that I should not lose any more. I have also been harassed by a doctor for being fat – he didn't know me before and it gave me a depressing couple of hours. All that, I thought, and *still*...

One woman, who has always seemed to need to assert that she is more powerful than I am, still refers to me as though I were very large. She, now, is three stone heavier than me, which is unprecedented and perhaps she does not like it. 'If you and I were shipwrecked', she said recently 'you would still be alive when the rescuers came whereas I would be dead.' She was referring to the fact that my fat stores would keep me from dying from lack of fuel and from hypothermia. Can she really not have noticed that she is now considerably larger than me?

But I suppose that's the point. Because I feel better about myself at this size my sense of self is much more intact. That makes me more powerful because I am not cowed out there in the world as I was before. And perhaps some people can't take that.

The last two and a half years have been tough going and it will continue to be so. It may even get tougher as my body fights to regain its lost self. Would I recommend it? Only if you really really want to lose weight, are prepared to make a lot of sacrifices and are willing to take on this regime for life. If so I recommend it with my heart, soul and body!

There have been many bright moments in this journey. Three in particular stand out:

Running for a bus in Princes Street in Edinburgh. Seeing the bus coming, knowing that I *could* catch it, taking off hand in hand with my husband and legging it along the pavement to get there in time. Breathless and exhilarated!

Going to the BBC to take part in one of the radio debates on weight. The nice studio manager said to me afterwards 'How did you get involved in this subject? You're not fat.' I am ashamed to say that my first thought was that he was sending me up. But he was so very pleasant; one of those transparent, honest, thoroughly good guys. I was confused at first. But on telling a friend she said 'No, of course he wasn't. You *aren't* fat now.' (I am, of course.)

Turning up at the doctor's surgery for an appointment the other day. The receptionist said 'Name, please.' Funny, I thought she knew me. I gave my name. 'Oh, my God,' she said. 'I *am* sorry. I didn't recognise you, I honestly didn't. You've lost so much weight.'

I don't feel a sense of triumphalism about this, just pleasure and achievement. The feeling of achievement comes not from the reduced weight *per se*, but from having stuck at something that was very difficult.

This does not mean that weight loss is for everyone. You have to be in the right emotional place for it. I was lucky; I was there. Not everybody is.

Now I feel I don't want to lose what I've gained by regaining what I've lost.

Part 2
How to Lose Weight and Keep It Off For Ever

Chapter Seven
How Not to Lose Weight

At some point in the early nineties it became apparent to those two great bastions of weight prejudice, the medical profession and women's magazines, that diets don't work. Ever since dieting was invented in the nineteenth century by a physician called Banting its built-in obsolescence factor was proved over and over again by the fact that it was never something people did only once. You went on a diet. You lost weight. You stopped the diet. You regained the weight – and more. This was the beginning of the familiar yo-yo cycle, the despair of dieters everywhere.

In an attempt to offer people weight loss that would be effective and permanent, health professionals and health editors began to come up with non-diet solutions. 'How to lose weight without dieting' became a ubiquitous cover-line on magazines and subtitle in books. The idea was that the jaded dieter, worn out and cynical with years of failed attempts to lose weight – or rather, to keep the weight off – would seize on this as a born-again method that this time would work.

The World Health Organisation issued some common-sense guidelines: eg that weight loss should be slow in order to be both effective and safe and not more than 2 lbs per week should be lost. This is sound: the body cannot burn more than a kilo of fat a week. If you lose more you are losing fluid or muscle. Fluid is usually lost at the beginning of a diet, which is why the first week's loss is often dramatic (though not a true weight loss). Losing lean tissue – muscle – is dangerous. Muscle loss leads to weakness and a decline in fitness. In fast weight-loss diets, heart muscle can be lost, leading to sudden death from heart attack. There have been many recorded incidents of such deaths where the true circumstances are covered up and attributed to the dieter's obesity – another case of blaming the fat person for everything.[1] But in these cases the heart attack has occurred when a substantial amount of weight has been lost; the hapless dieter was doing the very thing that society and the medical profession demanded.

To say that diets don't work is a fair statement if 'diet' is defined as an eating strategy with a beginning and an end. If a diet has a name – the Grapefruit Diet, the Two-Day-Diet, the 35-Plus Diet – it is very unlikely to be a way of eating you are going to be able to stay on for life. The figures for recidivism remain depressingly constant: 95–98 per cent of all weight lost is regained, plus some more. So what to do if you want to lose weight and keep it off? First beware of the the traps!

Some Weight-loss Myths

The Healthy Eating Fallacy

'How can I lose weight if diets don't work?' This was a question I put to a number of health professionals and obesity experts when I was writing *The Forbidden Body*.[2] The answer, they claimed, was actually simple. All I had to do was 'eat healthily'. Well, I've never eaten particularly unhealthily, but I thought I'd clean up my diet so that 'bad' foods didn't get a look in. 'Don't restrict quantity or calories', advised one expert. 'But promise yourself that the only food you give yourself will be of high quality. Nothing instant or processed, no convenience foods. Eat wholemeal bread, whole-grain cereals, brown rice – plenty of complex carbohydrates, lean meat, fish, fresh vegetables and fruit. Don't deprive yourself. Don't stint on puddings, but make sure they are made of good, wholesome ingredients. Don't drink fizzy drinks with aspartame – they give your brain the wrong signals and induce a craving for sweet things.'

I set to with a will. I actually love that kind of food, always eat wholemeal in preference to white bread, brown rice instead of white. I would prefer to binge on fruit than sweets and I would always choose a starter and a main course over a main and a pudding. I was already halfway there! I got quite fanatical about it.

It's a good feeling, concentrating on eating the food that is best for your body, knowing that if your diet is rich in anti-oxidants those disease-inducing free radicals are galloping round your bloodstream, will probably be zapped before they can do any harm. It's satisfying to know that your fruit and vegetable consumption is nearer to eight portions a day than the WHO's five a day recommendation. And you can feel quite smug when dried figs are your first choice for a real treat and you'd actually prefer them to cake. I wasn't deprived. I wasn't dieting. I was 'eating healthily' – the new recommendation for weight loss.

The pointer on the scales never budged. I had been conned.

A typical healthy eating day in my former life
Breakfast: Bowl of home-made muesli with prunes and natural yogurt. Slice of wholemeal toast, jam, no butter. Large glass of fruit juice.

Mid-morning: Snack of dried fruit, glass of fruit juice.

Lunch: Tuna salad with beans, olive oil dressing, couscous with pine nuts, wholemeal roll. Piece of fruit. Large glass of fruit juice.

Tea: Few dried apricots, glass of fruit juice.

Supper: Avocado with vinaigrette. Pasta with pesto, parmesan and roast vegetables or a delicious, healthy nut roast. Green salad with French dressing. Large glass of fruit juice. Fresh fruit salad with natural yogurt.

Great for maintaining the high weight I was then. But there was no way in the world I could have lost weight on that diet. Muesli is one of the healthiest, highest calorie foods there is. So is dried fruit. So is fruit juice. And avocados. And olive oil, included because it is also one of the health-giving substances and because some fat is necessary in the diet, is pure calories. I also love that health-food shop bread that is stuffed with nuts and seeds – about 300 calories a slice. I could eat fresh fruit and of course I do. I included dried fruit in that menu because it is one of my particular passions. Fat free but calorie dense and absolutely hopeless on a diet except in small quantities.

During that time, before the onset of ME, I took moderate exercise and my weight remained stable for years. Stable weight is the proof that your diet is calorifically right. If you're eating too much, you'll gain and if you are not taking in sufficient calories to match your energy expenditure, you'll lose weight. The body's natural state is to be in balance so that weight does not constantly dip and rise.

Many, many people who have gained weight as a result of emotionally generated chaotic eating reach a point, as I did, where they learn how to eat well. When this happens, the cycles of bingeing and starving cease. Habits like constant snacking or continually eating for comfort gradually disappear. The weight yo-yo stops – and this is where you are doing your body a huge favour. But that is the whole point about healthy eating: it is meant to stabilise you. Your body learns that famine is no longer around the corner. Eating healthily means eating enough and if you eat enough you will not lose weight because your body will have no need to feed upon itself.

Healthy eating – concentrating on good, whole foods and suppressing the starvation response – is an essential stopping-off post between years of disordered eating and deliberately trying to lose weight for the last time. Permanent weight loss should not be attempted as part of a continuum of failed diets. There has to be a resting time first, during which the body and mind can relax from the state of permanent hyperalertness which repeated dieting induces. If you cannot remember the last time your weight remained constant for more than a few months then ideally you should embark on a healthy eating plan that will stabilise it for about a year. It's a good idea to take a course of high-potency multivitamin and mineral pills too as it is likely that you have been lacking some essential substances.

This stage is also important if you have been a yo-yo dieter, because eating enough good food is the only way it will lose its power over you. It will re-educate your mind and your palate. Gradually your body will forget those feelings of desperation. Hunger and thirst are our most primitive impulses and the most powerful: once stirred into a state of life-saving readiness, they take some time to quieten. So while healthy eating as a way of losing weight is a fallacy, don't dismiss it as a way of life.

The Low-fat Fallacy

This is rather like the Healthy Eating plan. Fat is calorie dense. The WHO recommends that women on a normal diet (about 2000 calories) should aim to eat about 70 grams of fat per day; the requirement for a balanced diet. So if you cut that down – say to 20–30 grams of fat per day – you should lose weight. Right?

Wrong. And yet so many people swear by the low-fat solution. But even though low-fat eating is made easy for us by manufacturers who respond to the trend by producing reduced-fat butter, margarine, cheese and just about every kind of food you can buy – even reduced-fat chocolate – the obesity rate keeps climbing and the weight-loss failure rate stays about the same. It is extraordinary how much faith is invested in this as a solution, based on the erroneous belief that fat in your food transmutes to fat in your body.

Low-fat eating has become a religion with rules, rituals and sacrifices. We treat dietary fat as though it were the devil himself. Fat, we have been told, will give us heart attacks and make us fat. It's a given, surely?

I thought so until I started reading the research. There's too much of it to go into in depth here so I'll just give you two overviews. An article in *Science Magazine* entitled 'The Soft Science of Dietary Fat' stated that:

> Mainstream nutritional science has demonised dietary fat, yet 50 years and hundreds of millions of dollars of research have failed to prove that eating a low-fat diet will help you live longer.[3]

And Meir Stampfer, professor of epidemiology and nutrition at Harvard, said:

> People have got the wrong message that fat is bad. They have the mistaken assumption that if you eat fat, you get fat, but it is not the case that a low-fat diet will lead to a low-fat person.[4]

What you do have to beware of – and you won't hear this from any of the low-fat gurus – is not getting *enough* fat in your diet. Not only is too little fat deleterious to physical and mental health but it can actually prevent you from losing weight.

All cell membranes are made of lipoprotein, ie built of fat. If you don't have enough or the right sort of fat, you will make faulty membranes. A chronic shortage of dietary fat or repeated episodes of low-fat intake (as in yo-yo dieting) results in imperfect cell membranes due to lack of the right raw materials. In building terms, it's a 'no bricks' situation. These cell walls become leaky, causing the inappropriate passage of substances that should not pass from one cellular compartment to another. Consequently, certain chemical processes that should be taking place are halted and the calories which should be used in running those processes are not burnt up. It produces a similar situation to that when your metabolism goes into 'conserve' mode due to a low-calorie diet and you may actually gain weight.

You need essential fatty acids (efas) to make sure you have the membranes and the cellular architecture for metabolism to take place. If you don't eat enough dietary fat your body will try to manufacture efas from sugar. This means blood sugar levels will fall and you will feel very hungry.[5]

Essential fatty acids are found in natural oils and fats but not in packaged, processed food. These have the efas removed because they go rancid very quickly, reducing the product's shelf life. The fats in these products will be rubbish. But Udo Erasmus, a biochemist at the University of British Columbia in Vermont, has established that an intake of oily fish, olive oil and other vegetable oils raises the body's 'thermostat', causing more energy to be burnt. The efas in these oils and fats actually convert food into energy by transporting oxygen to the body's tissues. Oxygen burns fat and prevents it from being stored as body fat.[6]

Dr Susan Jebb, whose life's work is researching obesity, has said 'If I had to put my money on an area which is going to throw up some exciting information about obesity, it would be the role of fatty acids.'[7]

Too little fat in the diet can cause depression, aggression, irritability and hyperactivity. There can be serious neurological problems. And you won't look good, either – the skin gets very rough. It stands to reason. Skin cells, like all other cells, are made from lipoprotein. In other words, fat![8]

The gallbladder contains bile, which digests fats. If not enough fat is eaten the bile will sit there stagnating and this will encourage the formation of gallstones.

In one American study, obese patients were put on a 500-calorie per day low-fat diet. Before they began it, they were checked for signs of gallbladder disease: there was none. After eight weeks on the diet, 25 per cent of the subjects had developed gallstones.[9]

Apart from all these potential hazards, the essential vitamins A, D, E and K are fat soluble, unlike the others which are water soluble. If you don't have enough fat, the vitamins will pass right through and there will be a shortage.

There is a good reason for eating a diet *relatively* low in fat and that is the calorie content of fat compared to that of protein and carbohydrate. A gram of fat contains about 9 calories; protein or carbohydrate both contain about 4 calories per gram. So with the latter you get, as it were, more for your money – or calorie allowance. You can eat more food. If, for example, you are on a calorie allowance of 1700 per day, then a 300-calorie piece of chicken or fish, or a 300-calorie serving of rice or bread will give you more quantity than a 300-calorie piece of cheese.

If you cut your fat to about 30 per cent of your total *calorie* intake per day (not 30 per cent in weight) you should find you are satisfied. So on a diet of 1700 calories, about 30 per cent would give you 50 grams of fat. For those who habitually eat low-fat food, 50 grams will sound an enormous amount. It is 450 calories. If you feel you are not getting sufficient quantity of food, you could drop the fat content to 30–35 grams per day.

Most diets are based on a calorie allowance that is far too low. That is why 50 grams of fat – 450 calories – would use up too great a part of your allowance on such a regime. If you are following a more realistic diet, one which gives you sufficient calories, you should be able to incorporate a reasonable amount of fat. This means you don't miss out on the healthy fats in nuts, seeds and oils, though you will only eat them in small quantities.

If you don't eat enough fat you will feel hungry and you will experience cravings as your body tries to tell you what it needs. It is possible to eat a diet that is sufficient in energy (calories) and yet still feel hungry because you desperately need fat. Fat is satisfying; it has a high satiety value. You don't need a great deal of it, but insufficiency can have you prowling round the kitchen feeling pretty desperate without knowing what it is you lack.

Women tend to count the fat grams in everything, often using as a basic premise the belief that if they can get through the day having consumed *no* fat, it will be a day well spent. They feel great surges of satisfaction when they read the nutritional information on something and find that after 'fat' it says 'trace' or '0.3 grams'. I know. I used to do it. I would aim to get through a day having consumed about 10 grams of fat and I was not alone by any means. This, by the way, was when I was *not* losing weight. It was when I was following the dictum that if you eat a healthy diet that is low in fat you will get thinner. Like everything else it works only if the reduction in fat consumption means an overall calorie reduction.

Rosemary Conley says uncompromisingly that 'If you're trying to lose weight don't have olive oil. It makes you fat.'[11] One tablespoon of olive oil contains about 125 calories. A few of those in a week is not going to make you fat as long as you keep within the 30 per cent intake figure. It is unnecessary to ban good foods from your diet as though they were like some kind of bad fairy with 'I will make you fat' properties! Sugar will make you fat if you eat too much of it – *lettuce* will make you fat if you overdose!

Olive oil is good for you. And – heresy coming up – saturated fats are not the villains of the piece: 'trans' fats are. If you eat a moderate amount of natural saturated fat it will do no harm. So you can have butter on your bread (just count it in to your daily allowance). Natural products like butter contain the beneficial 'cis' fats.

The fat to avoid is hydrogenated fat. This is a process that solidifies oils, and produces harmful transfatty acids, so avoid all those margarines and spreads that are supposed to be so good for you. Do you really want to eat something that might contain butylated hydroxyanisole, tert-butylhydroquinone, disodium guanylate, 35trimethlhexanal, propyl octyl or dodecyl gallate? And that's only a few of the chemicals added to that nice yellow spread with the bucolic illustration on the box.[12]

At least two meals of oily fish a week will provide the efas you need, and if you have been on a low-fat regime for some time you will need to take Omega 3 supplements for your body to make up the deficiency. Rosemary Conley's recommendation of one serving of salmon per week is not sufficient.

So, while *lower* fat eating is recommended for health it will not, *per se*, hasten weight loss.

The Gym Fallacy

Going to the gym is the new religion. Like going to church, it is regular and ritualistic and people don't feel properly cleansed unless they've been. I took part in a radio programme after the

National Audit Office's pronouncement on the cost of obesity to the nation,[13] and I ended up saying exasperatedly that the government should close down all the gyms!

The reason for my frustration was that people believe that the gym is the Holy Grail of weight-loss solutions, just as they once believed that certain mad diets were. But like mad diets, gym workouts can be over the top, unrealistic and short term.

What happens is this. You take out gym membership in a spirit of enthusiastic resolve. Possibly you have read about yet another celebrity's huge weight loss; amazed, you look at the before and after pictures and you discover that it was Going to the Gym that did it. It's very seductive, especially if you read about broadcaster Anne Diamond, who said she didn't even have to diet, not really, it was all due to the hours put in at the gym. No one relishes the idea of cutting down on their food so if there's another way to lose weight, let's go for it!

It isn't only that. Somehow the collective thought processes of the nation have been channelled into the firm conviction that you cannot lose weight without going to the gym. This belief came about through the exhortations directed at us from various government and health bodies, to get up off our backsides and exercise. So unfamiliar is the population with the notion of moving their bodies in the time-honoured ways – walking, cycling, rushing around (on foot) – that the only route to exercise seems to be the road to the gym. And people usually drive there! It's the grown-up woman's equivalent of my daughter's pronouncement, when – aged two – she was whining to be picked up: 'What do you think you've got legs for?' said her grandfather. 'Putting tights on,' shot back Jane.

My exasperation on that phone-in programme came from the callers' blind insistence that the *only* way they could get some exercise was to go to the gym. As the 'expert' on the programme, I was presented with such problems as 'I don't have time to go to the gym' or 'I can't afford gym membership'. I began to sound like a cracked record. 'You don't need to go to the gym, all you need to do is walk briskly. Anywhere. It doesn't cost anything and it only need take about half an hour a day.' My responses were met with a certain amount of bewilderment. The callers, representing those who were either stung by or smug about the National Audit Office's report, which claimed (highly erroneously) that obesity costs the country around £2¹/₂ billion pounds per annum, were trying to demonstrate that their intentions to prevent or cure the curse of overweight were of the noblest order. And I was saying 'Don't bother'.

Going to the gym is like embarking on a diet. It will certainly help you lose weight and if you put in several hours a week of good solid working out, you will probably lose a great deal of weight fairly quickly. Then you will feel ecstatic and possibly you will increase your time at the gym in order to lose more weight. Amazing how it just falls off you, especially if combined with a calorie-controlled diet. I know a number of people who have lost weight this way. And put it back on again.

It is not a natural way to live. The gym carves out great chunks of your time. It's a slog to get there, get changed, get working out. The initial enthusiasm wears off. It's expensive. All in all, it's a pretty heavy commitment and most people don't stick to it. And like not sticking to a diet, the moment you backslide, the weight comes piling on again.

At least one study has demonstrated that periods of high-intensity activity are actually counterproductive. When the activity levels of people taking low-, moderate- and high-intensity exercise were measured, it was found that only those taking moderate exercise, such as walking and cycling, actually increased their overall energy expenditure. Those who undertook high-intensity activity, such as gym workouts, did not increase their total energy output because they compensated by being less active the rest of the time. The results were borne out by studies on obese patients which showed that 'adding exercise to an energy-restricted diet does not further increase weight loss because the costs of the extra activity are compensated by a reduction of energy spent on physical activity outside the training sessions.'

The proportion of time distributed between activities of low and moderate intensity is what influences the total energy expenditure,' concluded Klass Westerterp, who conducted the study at Maastricht University. In addition he points out that 'Moderate-intensity activities are better tolerated than high-intensity activities, especially by the middle-aged or obese.'[14]

So – on yer bike. If you want to join a gym join one for pleasure. Don't try to make it part of a weight-loss plan because you will be dependent on it and the chances that you will lapse are very high indeed.

The Fitness Video Fallacy

In theory this should work wonders. Aerobic exercise definitely assists weight loss and is also an important part of being in general good health. Like the gym, aerobics classes can be a bind, too much of a commitment for those who lead very busy lives. But to do the same thing in your own home, standing in front of your television – well, surely we can all manage that? We can tailor the routine to our own time and convenience, make it as vigorous as we choose, vary it from day to day. The possibilities are endless. Relatively cheap and trouble free, too.

There is an enormous range of videos to choose from. You can have standard, serious aerobic workouts presented by qualified instructors. Or – and these are the ones that sell – you can buy one presented by a diet guru, like Rosemary Conley, or a celebrity with a much-publicised weight loss.

Carol Vorderman and Vanessa Feltz, who are the slimmed-down women in the news at the time of writing, have both brought out exercise videos. People are seduced by these because they are excited by the success of the proponents and believe that if they follow the same regime they will reap the same rewards.

Fitness videos can work. If you spend upwards of 20 minutes a day in front of one, faithfully copying the apparently effortless instruction, you will raise your metabolic rate and burn calories. But for most people they are a nine-day wonder. They're quite fun to start with; there is music, something to watch and a feeling of achievement when you've finished it. But after a while they get boring. You can feel a bit of a prat standing in your living room prancing about in front of the telly. Then you miss a day, your resolve weakens – or you simply forget to do it. Or the day has passed and you haven't fitted in your routine. It can be particularly difficult if you have a family or housemates who also want the living room and the TV, not to mention the fact that they are likely to laugh themselves silly at the sight of you. The number of people who own fitness videos is enormous – they are huge sellers, like diet books. But like diet books, after the first flush of enthusiasm, most languish on a shelf.

I swore I would never buy one of the things, but Rosemary Conley gave me one of hers. I did try it, out of interest and curiosity. I quite enjoyed it even though I had great difficulty with right and left and kept falling over my own feet. It quickly palled and I went back to walking. And dancing.

If you've got the discipline, fitness videos are good. But I've yet to meet someone who has permanently incorporated them into their lifestyle.

The Pitfalls of Goal-oriented Weight Loss

When you've been overweight for a long time, it is difficult to find the impetus for change. You exist with it in a kind of tunnel, feeling that 'one day...' Some people are goaded into weight loss by a remark made to them. It is quite astounding what people feel free to say. One friend, meeting an acquaintance she hadn't seen for some time, was happily exchanging family news. Then the other woman leaned forward conspiratorially and whispered 'Did you *know* you've put on a lot of weight?' My friend was flabbergasted and furious, but where weight is concerned it was ever thus. People feel free to make the most insulting or personal remarks to someone they consider has 'a weight problem'.

While this sort of behaviour can be the spur that makes some people resolve to lose weight, by far the biggest motivator is The Goal. This can be imposed, as in the case of a doctor or surgeon insisting on weight loss before treatment or surgery is carried out. The psychological basis for this is hardly disposed to bring about success; resentment is likely (and justified) and there are ugly undertones of blackmail about it. Most people who attempt this kind of weight loss manage to lose some of the amount they are told to, but invariably put it back on. Losing weight because someone tells you that you must is being reduced to childlike status and recidivism is likely as a form of unconscious defiance.

But there is also the lure of the goal you set for yourself: the holiday, the wedding, the big event that you want to look your best for. It's not difficult to start a weight-loss plan when one of these occasions is forthcoming.

It goes like this: you book a holiday, perhaps six or even twelve months hence. You feel too ashamed to be seen in a swimsuit or with bare arms; you imagine that with a thinner body everything that the holiday has to offer will be more enjoyable. So you join a slimming club or buy a diet book and you start to lose weight, forever keeping that goal in mind. The goal itself provides the will power and you feel invincible. You can lose weight!

You can be even more focused if you're planning a wedding, especially if it's your own. At no other time in your life will you feel more on show. You might also want to lose weight before becoming pregnant in the belief that if your weight is lower at the start of pregnancy it will maximise the chances of both you and the baby being healthy throughout – though the evidence for this is flimsy.

The reason why actresses, models, television presenters and other women in the public eye have more success than most in keeping their weight down is that their lives are a series of recurring goals. There's nothing quite like being the focus of attention to concentrate the mind. But most of us live in relative obscurity and, even if friends or family goad us about our weight, it is not the same as appearing in front of millions of spectators, including journalists who will gleefully seize upon a couple of pounds a celebrity gains and trumpet it to the nation.

Belinda's Story

In spring 1984 the media were full of the story of Belinda Charlton, a glamorous, blonde 37-year-old who was in town to run her first London Marathon. Two years previously, Belinda had weighed 22 stone and could hardly get out of her chair. Now she was 12 stone lighter and running the Marathon; the media could not get enough of her phenomenal story, which she told in her autobiography *Big Is Invisible*.[15]

> One afternoon I sat, a tin of biscuits and a bottle of pop beside my chair, in front of the television, watching the London Marathon. More than anything I envied the competitors the energy and self-discipline necessary to run over 26 miles. The people on my screen were not super-athletes, but ordinary people running for fun, for a sport; for the dedicated few it was a way of life. I had never run, or done anything athletic, but used to love walking in the forest.

The running I watched on television seemed an escape, a freedom, like a kite or a bird soaring.

Belinda's stepson was running in the Marathon she watched and afterwards she told him she thought it was 'a marvellous achievement'. He suggested what, to Belinda, seemed a preposterous idea: that she should have a go and that he would train her. She was intrigued though and after reading a couple of books on running she began to believe it might be the cure for her overweight and depression. 'Running was an escape route... There were rewards: the feeling of achievement, pride, self-satisfaction and a new self-respect, a driving force to take me through the hard training months to the ultimate goal of the London Marathon.'

At first Belinda could only walk fairly short distances. Her first attempt at running lasted 30 seconds and left her with pounding heart, rasping breathing and legs like jelly – a far cry from the prospect of a marathon. But it was the start of a regime which was to make her feel increasingly good, physically and mentally, and which furnished the will power for her to diet.

A few months later, Belinda was able to take part in a three-and-a-half-mile Fun Run. She was walking, running and swimming every day with iron discipline. And she was dieting. Not surprisingly, she lost around six stone in seven months. Then she went to Israel. Early on in her month's holiday she trod on a sea urchin and was unable to run. She also abandoned her diet. If ever proof were needed that the dieted body will take its revenge as soon as you dare relax, Belinda received it. After only four weeks she had put on a stone and a half. And there, on her return home, lay her acceptance. She had been chosen for one of the sought-after places in the London Marathon; out of over 100,000 applications only 20,000 could be accepted.

She knew she had to do something drastic. She got in touch with her local television company. 'My acceptance for the London Marathon was special news, they might consider it qualified for the theatre of the absurd. I phoned and got an immediate response.'

TVS (now Meridian) responded by saying they would like to send a film crew round for the first of a series of programmes. Belinda now had a double goal: to lose weight to run the Marathon and to have a large TV audience watch her do so:

If the news of my acceptance for the Marathon had thrown me off balance the imminent arrival of the television crew meant there was no turning back. No more backsliding or I would make a public exhibition of myself. I would be doing that anyway, but to expose myself as too weak for my own good would be humiliating. People would probably laugh at the idea of me running a marathon in any event. But why not me? This was my chance to escape once and for all from my old flab-ridden world and to do so in front of the cameras. Maybe it would help me, a powerful monitor to prevent backsliding. I might even give hope to the thousands of others, who were the victims of their own ravenous appetites; who were obese and hopeless.

Television makes you feel very very special – while you're flavour of the moment, that is. Belinda's experience demonstrates this. Of that first programme, she said 'The biggest bonus of all was being the centre of attention for five solid hours... While this was happening they laughed at my jokes and apparently listened to my slightest comment. After years of unimportance and invisibility it was a heady experience.'

The day after the programme aired gave Belinda a taste of what was to come:

People came up to me and wished me well. I got free carrier bags for my shopping and the bank clerk did not look up my account on the computer when I presented a cheque for cashing. He just smilingly handed over the money. I was given a reduction in my taxi fares, I got served out of turn in a shopping queue, shopkeepers did not always want to see my cheque card when paying by cheque and I got served with great ceremony in restaurants... People phoned me, wrote to me and stopped me in the streets.

With that kind of visibility, considerably magnified, it is perhaps no wonder that celebrities feel they have an inescapable incentive to keep their weight down. For Belinda fame was the spur. What was more, the television company, mindful of the possible risk to a very overweight woman tackling such a task, put Belinda in the hands of a professional trainer. He devised a gruelling fitness regime and a tough diet for her, on which she aimed to lose 3–5 lbs per week. The weight fell off and before long she was running 50 miles a week.

So long as my progress was followed on television every two weeks there was an added incentive to do well. But I was also aware of the price I had to pay for this vanity. My success would be publicly acclaimed, but any faltering on my part, any suspicion of faint heart, would be publicly exposed. Sometimes, usually after a television show, failure seemed a remote possibility, like an accident that always happens to other people.

Just before the Marathon, the attention Belinda was attracting reached its height. The television company filmed a special pre-race party at her home. She was surrounded by family, friends and strangers and her confidence could hardly have been greater. In *Big Is Invisible* she continues her story:

During the party a photographer from the *Daily Mail* came to take my photograph. The next day the *Daily Mail* carried a double-page spread of me sitting in the garden by the river in running shorts. Overnight my story went national, and then even international. The following day the *Sun* also ran a double-page spread and then the story ripples spread. The phone went berserk. I was offered two film parts, both pornographic! I was asked to do photographic modelling, some of it respectable. I had to laugh at the demand for my body which had never been thought of very highly before...

There were offers to appear on television, write magazine articles, make personal appearances, open things and endorse products. I even got some passionate love letters from fans, and now everybody was recognising me in the street. I was a popular newsworthy package and I was loving every minute of it.

Belinda ran the Marathon and completed it. What had seemed an impossible, even risible goal two years before, became solid reality. 'At that moment,' she said, 'I was probably the most visible woman in London, my image transmitted by television throughout the world. It was a spectacular ego trip.'

The high of her achievement lasted for Belinda well after that first marathon. Losing so much weight had transformed her and she looked back on the woman she had been, finding it hardly credible that she had weighed 22 stone and been barely able to move. The following year she ran her second London Marathon, attracting the same level of publicity: this time with the publication of her autobiography. The excitement was still there, and there was also a reflective, quiet confidence as she reviewed the past three years: 'I know I could not have lost the weight without the running and could not have run the Marathon without losing weight. Now that the weight is off, I know I can keep it off as long as I run regularly and eat sensibly.'

Belinda Charlton had a good deal more than the transient fifteen minutes of fame. After the second marathon she was still much in demand. I was working for the BBC at the time and was sent to interview her. Because of her personality – which was sparky and positive – and her incredible determination, I felt sure that she would be one of the 5 per cent who kept the weight off.

That was in 1985. In 2000, I saw Belinda again. She had regained most of the weight but not within two years as do the majority of dieters. The figure at which weight loss is considered to be permanent is five years. Belinda put her weight back on after six.

It crept up gradually at first, not a great deal, just a stone or so. She had stopped dieting. Even so, she didn't worry. She thought she had found the secret: that as long as she ran she would not become very overweight. But one day, out running, she developed shooting pains in her feet. It was the curse of many runners: arthritis. She had to stop running. She told me:

That was the beginning of the end. Everything went to pot. I was a bit sorry for myself but I got a nice new job in public relations. I was overweight by then but I was not being treated badly in the way that you can be in that business, so everything was going very nicely. But the weight kept going on. I didn't worry. I told myself to forget about it. But you look at other women and realise that they don't look like you. They were zipping round London with their mobile phones and by then I was waddling round London.

In spite of not running, Belinda is still very active. Her job – putting on major corporate and charity events – requires a great deal of standing and rushing around. She swims regularly and walks about two miles a day. But Belinda has a severely dieted body, one which was just waiting for the chance to rebuild itself. And she has a problem with food. The seeds of her downfall are contained in a tiny paragraph in *Big Is Invisible* amid the euphoria of completing the Marathon and achieving the weight loss: 'My weaknesses are still there, not far beneath the burnished new surface. I yearn for all the fattening foods, sweets, cakes, biscuits and comfort snacks.'

She is fully aware of her problem. She said: 'I lack the mechanism that says I've had enough. Enough is not as good as a feast – a feast is always much better. I think food is like a drug. I believe the way you have to deal with it is the way that people do with any addiction. People say moderate your intake – that doesn't do it. Your main aim every day is just to get through that day without eating too much of the wrong things but it's rather pathetic that that's what you have to do. I can't leave anything on my plate.'

Now in her fifties, Belinda knew she had decisions to make. But the problem, she believed, was that she no longer had a goal to aim for. And she was in a dilemma.

I don't want to do it again. Life's too short. It's not worth all that agony, all that effort. And Warwick [her husband] will tell you what a bore I am. You know that you have to think about it all the time. You plan your day around the food. The thought of doing it again is such a nightmare and I think to myself, does it really matter? And I had been thinking, no, it doesn't matter. I can get on with life perfectly well, I don't need to have this aggravation. I'll try not to eat too much but I'm not going to think about it. There are other things I want to do that are more interesting than thinking about food all the time. But then you get to a point where you realise you're becoming disabled because you're too heavy. That you look ridiculous; it's hurting your life; it's damaging your career; you're not being taken seriously; you're that funny, fat woman and you think, why am I handicapping myself like this? People are very fattist; indeed I am myself. I know what it's like, you get tired, you can't do things as well as you could. I wouldn't employ people who are very fat, I know I wouldn't.

Gaining the weight back definitely affects my self-esteem. If you walk into a room you know you are drawn to talk to people who are attractive, so you know how people feel about you. If they do like you it's despite the weight. Sometimes you'll be talking to someone and you realise they're pitying you. People look at you and think about weight. They think, oh, my God, I could end up like her. They look at you and think, how are you going to affect me?

I couldn't go back to my original diet, which was low fat and low carbohydrate, just a bit of cottage cheese. I was starving. I don't know how I did it and I don't know why I can't even get an eighth of it off now. I suppose I haven't got a goal. Except that if I don't get the weight off now, I'm going to become an old woman. It could be a long life but one which is semi-handicapped – a self-inflicted semi-handicap.

Three months after our meeting, Belinda's knee 'gave way'. For five months she could not walk at all. It was a shock for someone who is always on the go and it made her rethink. Now, with her knee fully recovered, she is walking seriously every day.

'It's easy to feel encouraged when you find yourself getting fitter and achieving 100 per cent improvement in a week,' she says. 'When I'm walking regularly it's easier not to give in and eat a chocolate cake. So I'm back on a diet. I've lost a stone and a half and I feel a lot better. But what I won't be doing is going back to the way I lost weight before: the misery of starvation.'

Belinda's story illustrates one of the toughest things about losing weight: you can never go back. If the weight loss has come about through drastic exercise and diet, then that has to be the pattern for the rest of your life. For Belinda, running did it, and the Marathon was the goal that kept her iron resolve going for two years. No one can keep that up for life and her new, gentler exercise and diet regime is far more likely to result in permanent – though much slower – weight loss.

VLCDs

This stands for very low-calorie diets and refers to the Cambridge Diet, Slimfast, Optifast, Nutraslim and other meal-replacement diet drinks, soups or bars. They are not good news. You drink a protein- and vitamin-enriched shake two or three times a day instead of meals and lose weight very fast indeed. Your calorie intake will be around 500 a day, which is not enough for anyone.

Doctors sometimes argue that VLCDs are called for in cases where extreme obesity is at a life-threatening stage. I cannot see that fast weight loss can ever be beneficial. Besides, the body will be in such a state of deprivation and hyperacuity that as soon as you start eating real food again, back will come the weight plus a lot more for safety's sake.

There is an organisation called Obesity Lifeline, whose intentions are honourable but whose methods seem questionable. Operating in small groups led by counsellors, they put you on a VLCD for three months, claiming that food addiction is like alcoholism and the only way to conquer it is to banish food from the diet. During the three months, you are assisted in the process of discovering the emotional power food has over you and which foods are your particular downfall. Then the 'trigger' foods are introduced one by one until, the theory goes, you can deal with them without bingeing.

Jill Welbourne is opposed to VLCDs. I asked her what she thought of the methods used by Obesity Lifeline.

No food can lose its power over you if you're only eating 500 calories a day. I just don't believe that, you'd feel panicky and unsafe. It's like being in a concentration camp. It says famine, famine, famine. I can't help feeling this is a reincarnation of the Cambridge Diet. What about energy? You will have to sacrifice some metabolic processes that you would normally carry out because you haven't got the fuel to do it. It's rubbish to say you won't lose muscle at a rate of three stone in three months – that's half a pound a day and that's ridiculous. It's dangerous. The maximum you can safely lose in a week is a kilo and really it's better if it's less. They're losing 42 pounds when in that time I think you ought to lose no more than 20. They're losing twice as much as I think it is safe to lose.

There is a certain logic to the idea of withdrawing food altogether but it is flawed. Drawing a comparison between food addiction and alcoholism may not be helpful to the addict because, unlike alcohol, no one can cut food permanently out of their diet. Richard Atkinson, one of the scientists who discovered the virus said to be one cause of obesity, said 'It's like telling an alcoholic, "you must have three drinks a day, but you can't have any more." '[16]

The whole point about VLCDs is that they are such a deprivation to body and mind that the urge to binge increases a thousandfold for many people, just as it does after a period of starvation. While I recognise that food addiction is a real and devastating problem for many fat people, I do not believe that a drastic 500-calorie-a-day meal-replacement plan is the answer. Bar Hewlett, founder of Obesity Lifeline, lost six stone using this method and she has kept it off but she is very rare. There are exceptions to every rule.

Many people who enthusiastically embraced VLCDs in the eighties find that their metabolisms have been permanently impaired by their use. You cannot starve the body and expect it not to adopt drastic measures to stop you doing so again.

In clinical practice, Jill Welbourne has seen patients who have actually *failed* to lose any weight on a starvation diet. 'It's genetic, the ability to survive on nothing and therefore not lose weight because the body goes into extreme conserving mode. I had one patient who was eating one plum, half an orange and two bits of lettuce and tomato daily and not losing weight. There were witnesses that this was all she ate. She was low weight but she was a survivor – her body refused to let her lose any more.'

Apart from their inefficacy in long term-weight loss, VLCDs have been found to be extremely dangerous. Jill Welbourne explains why:

When you break down cells that fast you've got to be able to deal with the 'rubble' that's left. You can't just pull the wall down and leave the bricks lying there. But the calorie intake is too low to deal with those breakdown products. You need carbohydrate energy to do the biochemical 'clearing up'. If you're losing weight very fast you're breaking down muscle cells and releasing a lot of potassium but you haven't got sufficient energy for your kidneys to deal with it safely. The potassium gets into the circulation and unbalances your potassium/sodium relationship. This imbalance affects muscle cells and can lead to cardiac arrest.

Too many people have died from heart failure on VLCDs, particularly in the refeeding period after the diet.[17] Bar Hewlett says that this does not happen now because the protein in modern VLCDs is of better quality with all the necessary amino acids. But I am not convinced there is a place for these diets.

I could not cope with a regime that totally denied food and I know that 500–600 calories a day would make me feel terrible. But Obesity Lifeline clearly feel that for some people with addictive food problems, VLCDs are the way forward. If you are tempted, ask yourself what benefit you would gain. You might get a fast initial weight loss but you would also end up with a faulty metabolism, a body which panics if you let it get hungry and a whole lot of extra weight. Your purse will be lighter, your body heavier than ever and your mood will be black.

This is a matter of individual choice, however. If you have a problem with serious food addiction you may want to try Obesity Lifeline. Just make sure you read the research on VLCDs.

And Any Other Low-Calorie Diets...

Most of these come in books and magazines and can sound extremely persuasive. As a book reviewer, I get sent a great number of diet books which give me an opportunity to see what is really going on. Most of these books would do you more good if you tore them up and ate them. And most don't stay in print for long so that would seem to be proving something obvious.

But they can be very seductive, not least because they invariably have subtitles designed to make you think that a weight-loss diet is not only a necessary part of life, it is a deliriously happy, wonderful, desirable state of affairs, and pity the poor thin people who can't really afford to indulge in this behaviour...

These are a few of the subtitles of the diet books on my shelves:

- The on/off diet that puts the fun back into losing weight
- Eat as much asyou like and still lose weight
- The no-hunger, luxurious weight loss plan that really works
- The perfect diet for those who love food
- How to lose weight permanently without dieting
- The revolutionary new diet for the nineties
- Lose weight without cutting calories

- How to lose weight and never gain it back
- Up to one pound weight loss per day

Diet peddlers – and that includes the authors of diet books –
will try anything to lure the consumer. For instance, have you
heard of 'sexy dieting'?[18] Well, get to it, if your sex life is not all
you'd like it to be! Sexy dieting admonishes that 'being touched is
only good if you can feel it, so your fat layer must be thin.' (Can't
say I know anyone whose fatness has been a barrier to sexual
satisfaction.) You might also like to know that if you have been
eating 'stodge, cakes and sweets' you will be 'fat and soporific' – so
no sexy mood there, then. And do avoid the 'bloaters, which make
people look fatter than they are by swelling up inside the body.'
That means fizzy drinks, frothy lagers and dried food which needs
reconstituting with water. Imagine what this could do to the
massive Coca Cola industry if women knew that the product they
depend upon to keep them thin was actually making them look
fatter! My advice if you have shares in Coke would be to sell them
now before the word spreads. One beauty editor actually
recommends taking Rennie's Deflatine tablets.[19] God forbid that
women's stomachs should ever show signs of the curves that make
us female; out with the washboards!

The authors of these diets work very hard to think up a new
gimmick: not an easy task in an age where every other book
published seems to be about dieting. The gimmicks are actually
meaningless; inevitably they mask yet another low-calorie regime.

For instance, the On/Off Diet ('that puts the fun back into
losing weight') is actually called the Two-Day Diet.[20] The idea
behind this is – you've guessed it – that you have a day on the
diet and a day off. 'There are On Days to take the fat off – fast,'
runs the blurb. 'And Off Days – to provide the reward for a job
well done.'

Sounds like something you could stick to? The authors think so,
too. 'The *requirement* [their emphasis] to eat what you love on your
Off Days is the basis for the success of the Two-Day Diet.'

Unfortunately, most people will be drawn to the promise that it
will 'take the fat off fast' – three to five pounds a week, the book
claims, even though that should sound warning bells. The On
Days will give you around 700 calories. The Off Days are not off

days at all – you can have 1200 calories. Forget it. You'd lose weight fast, certainly – and then you'd put it all back on again.

The Rotation Diet[21] is a similar idea: you eat 600, 900 and 1200 calories. The author claims proudly that you will lose about a pound a day. This is utterly unsafe.

Then there is the new Blood Group Diet, which theorises that different foods suit different blood groups. This smacks of desperation. All the gimmicks have been used up so it's time to get really wacky.

What happens next is that the old chestnuts come back: the ones that were crazes until they were discredited, so they go away and lie down for a few years then rear their heads for a new generation of dieters.

The following is an absolutely typical tale of despair from Lee Kennedy, a very large, very dieted woman. Find me the fat woman who doesn't read it with a sense of 'I've been there' familiarity:

> I've done the usual weary slog through every imaginable diet over the years, and it's true, of course, the lard all comes back, increases and becomes harder to shift, every time – yet I *keep* doing it! As I grow older, I'm afraid of dying from some fat-related malady, but I'm equally sure that the kind of strict starvation diet I now have to resort to to lose even a little weight may be equally damaging. I once attended an NHS obesity clinic where I was put on a three-month blitz that whacked three stone off me. It involved a tablespoon of bran, an Oxo or some salty drink, and four quarts of skimmed milk a day (or three semi-skimmed) – nothing else, except perhaps some sugarless jelly and the vitamin supplements and Fybogel. I stuck to it, too.

There are many lessons here, not least of which is that it isn't just those with an eye to a pound or a dollar who peddle ridiculously low-calorie diets. Amazingly, in our so-called enlightened times, the medical profession is also rather fond of them, as Lee discovered at her obesity clinic. They will often talk about administering these diets under 'supervised conditions', perhaps in hospital, and they state that the crash diet is for those whose life is threatened by their weight. The fact that a very low-calorie diet is in itself life-threatening doesn't seem to be taken into consideration, nor does the fact that as soon as you start eating after this deprivation you *gain weight*!

The Magical Diet

The *Daily Mail* is particularly good at this. You'd think its readers would wonder why the paper would need to keep publishing new diets if they worked in the first place but no, around comes another one.

In the middle of writing this book, I received a phone call from a good friend. 'There's a diet in today's *Mail*', Annie announced. 'It sounds really good. You can eat bacon and bagels and baked beans. I think I should give it a go'.

I was taken aback. This friend, who is large and would like to lose quite a lot of weight, had previously recognised that for whatever reason, now was not the time for her to do it. Weight loss is one of those mysterious psychological processes; there comes a time when you think yes, I want to do it and I want to do it *now*. None of us knows why we didn't reach that stage two months or two years ago but, until it happens, there is no point in trying to lose weight. Only when the body and subconscious mind meet in agreement and let you know their decision will you be able to do it. And Annie and I had agreed many times that her time had not come.

Now, the diet in the *Daily Mail* had seduced her. Why? I wanted to know. She said that the *Daily Mail* was so aspirational it made her feel that perhaps she should be trying to be like the people in it. After all, the woman featured in the diet had lost three stone, had gone from a size 16 to a size 8 in eight months. It had sounded so easy. Maybe she should be trying to be one of the Beautiful People too.

Very clever: worthy of the most successful used-car salesman. I told Annie that the reason the diet allowed bagels and bacon was that it had calculated them into its daily calorie allowance. There's no magic, I told her. You can lose weight on chocolate.

Annie was not convinced. One day she said she had eaten four grissini (breadsticks) for lunch. Why not a bread roll? I asked. Much more nutritionally sound. The diet called for grissini, she replied. What's more the diet gave you a list of foods to buy before you started. Annie had bought every single one, including Branston Pickle. 'I hate Branston Pickle,' she wailed. 'What has happened to my mind?'

That's easy. She was under a spell, the Magic Diet spell. Now, as every child knows, spells only work if you follow them correctly, every step of the way. If Annie had not had grissini and Branston Pickle – well, she would not have lost weight, would she?

I looked at this diet. Based on Weight Watchers' points system it was pretty low calorie. ('I'm hungry all the time,' complained Annie halfway through the diet.) But it had magic people in it, like the Diet Psychiatrist (actually a nutritionist), the Exercise Expert and, of course, the Definitive Diet Agony Aunt. There was helpful, motivating advice from them each day of the diet. Like brushing your teeth so that the taste of toothpaste would stop you wanting to eat or drink anything. On Day Three the Diet Psychiatrist suggests that by now you will be experiencing withdrawal symptoms from the high-fat or -sugar foods you have eliminated. You will be feeling out of sorts and lacking energy.

This is not normal. It shows the diet is too low in calories: ie energy. Further evidence was to be found in the advice on Day Five: that at this stage it is common to be feeling irritable, restless, uptight, and suffering from headaches. This is perfectly normal, pronounces 'The Psychometer'. It isn't. If you are feeling like that you are not having enough to eat and you're not far from having a binge. 'I did have three Hob Nobs with my tea,' confessed Annie. I should think so too!

Halfway through the diet, Annie was waking in the night ravenously hungry. After four weeks she broke the diet and bought a box of cakes and a bar of chocolate. Her intellect knew all along that it wouldn't work but it held out such a tempting promise...

There are lots of Magic Diets around now. 'Do you wish you had a magic formula for losing weight and keeping it off? Well now you do,' announced a press release. This was for a book called *The Formula: The Sensational 40+30+30 Fat Burning Nutrition Programme.* (That's a diet to you and me.)

The thing about this one is that it is based on a sound principle: that you eat 40 per cent carbohydrate, 30 per cent fat and 30 per cent protein. So where's the magic? It must be in the Fat Flush

Formula, which is 'so dramatic that dieters often ask if they can stay on it indefinitely'.[22] This in itself would sell a lot of books.

And so on. Magic diets often come with fake medical credentials, which is extremely alarming because people then believe in them implicitly. A friend of mine, a trained nurse and health visitor, got very excited about a diet she'd started. It was very low calorie and contained bizarre things like Ritz crackers instead of bread. 'It's bound to be okay,' she said. 'It's produced by the British Heart Foundation.' I was taken aback and asked her to send me a copy. It was headed 'The Heart Institute Diet'. I checked and found there was no such organisation but my friend, disbelief suspended as invariably happens when in search of the Magical Diet, had subconsciously translated this bogus diet into something endorsed by the BHF and therefore bound to be not only effective but good for health.

The British Heart Foundation has never put its name to this kind of cranky, crash diet. It is not only mad, it is unsafe.

Drugs and Big Business

- Pill will make fat a thin [sic] of the past: scientists develop new wonder drug
- Mood Food: Scientists' scheme to add 'happy chemical' as aid to diet may end in mass mind control, critic fears
- Is this anti-depressant a new weight-loss drug?
- Gene therapy will banish fat for ever
- Danger drugs freely given to all who ask

So if not the Magic Diet, what about the Magic Bullet? Listed above is a very small selection of random headlines in my cuttings collection which show both the longing for the elusive magic bullet and the concerns voiced by a few responsible journalists. Drugs are the current fashionable weight-loss option, though they have been around in some form for over a century.

The medical profession is very keen on these drugs. I am convinced this is because they know they have nothing else to offer. People wanting to lose weight need sound nutritional advice and continuous support. The NHS has not invested in these resources; fat patients continue to ask their doctors for help, so what better solution than to send them away with a prescription? A bit like the treatment of depression, really.

There is also the tiny matter of the unbelievably vast sums of money to be made from the production of such drugs and the ethics of their availability are questionable. There are slimming clinics all over the country where you can buy yourself these products with a prescription from the attending doctor.

No, you don't have to be overweight to get the drugs. Numerous journalists without an ounce of spare flesh have written investigative pieces about slimming clinics. They have turned up and asked for a prescription and been given one. One example: Clare Thompson went to the Berkshire Diet Clinic wanting to reduce from a size 12 to a 10 (why? I have to ask rhetorically).[23]

She did not think she would get the pills. Her BMI was 24.1. In (totally unrealistic) fat police terms overweight officially starts with a BMI of 25. The doctor at the clinic asked her why she wanted to lose weight. She said she felt too fat. 'The media are terrible,' he said. 'They show pictures of skinny models and then accuse us of being irresponsible for prescribing these pills.'

Uh? Did he mean that he was *not* being irresponsible prescribing a powerful weight-loss drug with side-effects to someone whose size and BMI were normal even according to the draconian limits of the medical profession? Well, 'trust me, I'm a doctor'.

Then came Xenical (Orlistat), the drug which would make you thin by absorbing the fat you have eaten. How, you might wonder, will that help you lose weight when, as I hope I have demonstrated, you can actually gain or maintain weight on a virtually fat-free, actually 'healthy-eating' diet? You've guessed it: Xenical only works with 'Dietary Discipline'. You actually have to lose some weight before the drug can be prescribed, just to show that you can do it. And while taking Xenical you have to follow a calorie-controlled, low-fat diet. At the moment, you can take it for two years only, and a one-year trial showed the average weight loss to be 1st 7 lb. While losing weight that slowly is to be recommended, I question the use of a drug to do so.

Side-effects include such delights as diarrhoea and 'anal leakage'; weight-loss plateaus after a fairly short time. And why does no one seem to address the obvious question: if you follow the diet instructions issued when Xenical is prescribed, you'd lose weight anyway?

John Humphrys, that wonderfully feisty and waspish broadcaster, is sceptical about the real purpose of drugs like Xenical: 'Once again we have the drug company telling us this is not a lifestyle drug. It is for those who are clinically obese. Of course, of course. No doubt the company will fight like tigers to stop the pill being sold to those who want to buy it.'[24]

Only a few weeks after Xenical was licensed in Britain, Humphrys received a glossy leaflet offering him '...the new wonder drug for a very reasonable £110 for one month's supply or even better, £295 for three months. Plus post and packing, of course. How could I refuse? This, as the leaflet pointed out in its subtle way, was "the new slimming breakthrough for the millennium...available to you now!!"'[25]

As yet, Xenical has been 'safe', a word we have to use relatively in drug terms. But there have been other 'safe' weight-loss drugs which have now been withdrawn because people died from taking them. Fenfluramine, dexfenfluramine and fen-phen (fenfluramine combined with phentermine) were taken off the market after fatal side-effects occurred with their use: primary pulmonary hypertension and heart failure.

Julia Polak, a professor at the Hammersmith Royal Postgraduate Medical School in London, developed primary pulmonary hypertension and heart failure after taking a three-month course of fenfluramine. She was given an emergency heart-lung transplant.

She admits she took the pills out of vanity, wanting to 'look good in a bikini again after having a baby.' But she only had one or two pounds to lose. You have to question the prescribing of a weight-loss drug to someone who did not need it.[26]

The National Association to Advance Fat Acceptance (NAAFA) has a very clear policy on all these drugs. Though the organisation is speaking for America, surely the same must apply to the rest of the world:

Since weight-loss drugs fail to achieve permanent weight loss and can result in negative health consequences, since the governmental agency responsible for regulating weight-loss drugs has not protected consumers from dangerous weight-loss drugs, and since people taking diet drugs are rarely given sufficient information to allow them to give true informed consent, the National Association to Advance Fat Acceptance strongly discourages people of any size from taking drugs for the purpose of weight loss. Further, NAAFA condemns obesity researchers and drug manufacturers who profit from inadequately tested weight-loss drugs. In addition, because many consumers' motivation for weight loss is to escape size discrimination and weight-related social stigma and such motivation necessitates a political rather than medical response, and because health status can be improved independent of weight loss, NAAFA demands that the Food and Drug Administration denies approval of any weight-loss drug presented for approval that does not show clear health benefits apart from temporary weight loss.

Surgery

Surgery is for the desperate and I mean that quite literally. It is for those who genuinely cannot lose weight by dieting and whose lives are at risk through extreme fatness. Though SIZE and NAAFA do not endorse weight-loss surgery I have been persuaded that for some it is the only option.

I am persuaded by the fact that there are those who are so large that they risk death if they do not reduce their weight. These people do not have a death wish; if they could diet, they would. Their plight is terrifying.

But there are risks and horrible side-effects from weight-loss surgery. There are survivors' groups in America, Australia and Britain: people for whom surgery has been nothing but a bad thing.

My friend Caroline is the reason I think surgery has its place. She was 28 stone, disabled (not by her size), suffering from sleep apnoea and congestive heart failure and her prognosis was poor. She knew that if she did not lose weight she would almost certainly die within the next ten years and she was only 35. Caroline was opposed to surgical intervention but she had an intractable eating disorder of emotional origin and she was not in a position to limit her intake. In addition, her disability meant that she could do very little in the way of exercise.

When things became very grave indeed and Caroline could not even lie down because she could not breathe, she began to consider surgery. She was advised that any surgery at her weight and with her health problems was extremely risky. After many consultations and much waiting it was agreed that she should have a fairly new procedure, the gastric lap band.

This is the least invasive type of weight-loss surgery. It can be done, keyhole style, through a small incision. A doughnut-shaped band is placed around the top of the stomach, reducing its capacity to a few tiny spoonfuls. Through a port, placed under the skin, fluid is injected so the band is inflated and constricts the stomach. Fairly frequent tightening of this band is needed, necessitating a hospital visit each time.

Caroline was told that she had only a one in four chance of surviving the operation. Happily she did survive it and that was two years ago. She has lost three stone: not the vast weight loss that is generally touted with this kind of surgery but healthier for being slow. This is her account of the experience:

> I am sick every single day. You can only take very tiny amounts of food at a time and even a teaspoon too much will make you sick. Every time the band is tightened you have to learn all over again what you can and can't have. It isn't just quantity; you find that you need to eat different foods as well. I don't know why that is.
>
> I am in awful pain for much of the time. If the band is too tight you get a lot of heartburn. For a long time now I have had a lot of pain and sickness. I didn't know it would be like this. I'd heard about someone who had had the band and experienced no problems and lost loads of weight in a year.
>
> You can't have a social life because you just don't know when you are going to be sick.
>
> The band controls portion size but it doesn't help with the original problem with food. You can still eat things like cheese and chocolate. I can only lose weight by living in an environment where the food is totally controlled. It hasn't changed my relationship with food. I eat frequently to keep 'topped up' because I can't tolerate physical hunger. That's why I'm losing the weight slowly.

I'm still in conflict because my emotional issues with food haven't been resolved. I need the security of my weight around me. It's for protection. Mentally I want and need to be fat, but physically it was killing me. This operation was my only chance.

For anyone in a situation like mine, I would recommend this operation as long as they don't think it's going to work like magic. I would say don't expect it to change your relationship with food. If I had this band removed the weight would be back.

It is clear that Caroline had no other choice. I think her surgery was justified: she knew the risks and she was prepared to take them. Though the size-acceptance movement opposes surgery, I cannot see an alternative for people in her situation. And her particular operation is reversible. If she *were* to gain control of her eating and feel confident in maintaining her lower weight, the band could be removed, but Caroline does not think that this will happen. There is no place for political beliefs that do not take individual suffering into consideration. The size-acceptance movement opposes surgery as being mutilating and because it further pathologises the condition of fatness. I would agree, except in cases like Caroline's. NAAFA's position on weight-loss surgery is thoughtful and clear:

There is no conclusive evidence that gastrointestinal surgery for weight loss increases longevity or improves overall health. There are a tremendous number of deaths and severe complications associated with weight-loss surgeries. Since non-invasive treatments for comorbidity factors exist, the presence of comorbidity factors is not a valid justification for surgery. Therefore, the National Association to Advance Fat Acceptance condemns gastrointestinal surgery for weight loss under any circumstances. Until all weight-loss surgeries are discontinued, NAAFA urges that such surgeries be restricted to controlled studies conducted by trained medical researchers. Further, NAAFA believes that the psychosocial suffering that fat people face is more appropriately relieved by social and political reform than by surgery.

There are three basic types of weight-loss surgery: stomach stapling, gastric bypass and gastric lap banding. The last, which Caroline underwent, is the least available. There have been deaths with them all.

Professor John Baxter, one of the few UK surgeons to perform these operations, says that surgery has been found to be overwhelmingly better than drugs in improving quality of life. He favours the bypass operation, which I wouldn't touch with a bargepole and nor would Caroline. But he is, as far as one can see, non-judgmental: 'There seems to be an attitude that obesity is a self-imposed condition caused by lack of self-control. But it is a metabolic disease, like diabetes, and needs treating. Drug and genetic cures are still a long way off and there is absolutely no doubt that surgery offers the best hope for this group.'[27]

Fads and Scams

'Lose two pounds per day while you eat anything you want.' This is the heading on the publicity for a 'revolutionary' (always beware that word in connection with weight loss: it crops up a lot!) new product. This one is little tablets that you drop into your tea or coffee. Then the magic starts, for these contain the 'perfect combination of two fat eating agents... More than 3000 "fat eating" micro-elements are diffused in your drink. They are capable of devouring and eliminating up to four pounds of excess weight in 24 to 48 hours.'

This is not a miracle, continues the blurb sternly, because 'everything is based on extremely serious research.' You don't have to cut a single calorie, you just carry on eating as much as you want of whatever you want and your fat will just be consumed.

The most worrying thing about advertisements like this is that thousands and thousands of women believe them. The products are always immensely expensive but that is not a deterrent. The scams go on, not only because they cannot be regulated but because they are so profitable. They are profitable because women, often sane and otherwise intelligent women, think that they could work. Like the magical diet, these products offer a spell that will miraculously remove all that weight you don't want and it will be painless and easy.

Sadly, I know women who fall for these things; women who temporarily seem to take leave of their senses. Anything for the magic cure.

There are tablets. There are patches which will do anything from remove your appetite to remove your fat cells. There are creams to massage the fat away, wraps which will extract it through your skin, exotic vitamin or herbal extracts and a myriad other products.

The market is flooded with 'miracles' like this and it seems that there is no way to nail down and prosecute their touts. Our law has no teeth when it comes to catching the perpetrators. There are too many of them and they are too slippery. This is the reply I got from a trading standards officer about the proliferation of 'miracle' weight-loss products:

> Products that allegedly lead to weight loss may be subject to the Trade Descriptions Act if it can be shown that an advertisement is false or misleading to a material degree. Our main difficulty is proving falseness. The advertiser does not have to prove to us that their statement is accurate. We have to prove it is false beyond reasonable doubt and offends against a particular piece of legislation. In addition many of these advertisements are really just scams where it is particularly difficult to track down just who it is who is behind them. If someone is identified they will usually produce some documentary evidence that is difficult to verify before they wind the business up and disappear.[28]

The officer did not add 'laughing all the way to the bank' so I have. Sometimes these products appear under a veneer of respectability: they claim to be backed by research. I know a number of women who were seduced by Fat Magnets: a product made from chitosan, a 'naturally occurring shellfish fibre which has the ability to attract itself to fat' – a bit like a natural version of Xenical and without the side-effects.

Professor John Garrow, international obesity researcher and chairman of HealthWatch, conducted tests on Fat Magnets. If they were effective, he said, there should have been a lot of fat in the stools of those who were taking them. But there wasn't. Garrow stated that Fat Magnets 'are not an effective weight-loss remedy'.[29]

Nor, I can assure you, is anything else in the fads and scams category. There is nothing you can buy to cause weight loss.

Low-carbohydrate/High-protein/High-fat Diets

As I write, these are the fad of the moment, their selling power potentiated by the fact that they are apparently used by those Hollywood stars who have dieted from their gross size-10 bodies to a more acceptable size 4. The peddlars trade on a fashionable, new condition called 'insulin resistance'. Carbohydrate is what makes us fat, they say, so carbohydrate should be cut to a minimum because eating it causes too much insulin to be released.

It is extremely difficult to eat lots of protein and fat without carbohydrate, so these diets would almost certainly make you reduce your calorie intake. The body does burn calories more efficiently when you eat protein but too much protein is dangerous: it overloads the kidneys. Not so.

On these diets your body goes into a state of ketosis, which is not only bad for you, it's pretty unpleasant. You get nausea, bad breath and a nasty taste in your mouth.

Which?, the British consumer magazine, tested some of these diets and found they gave major cause for concern. *Dr Atkins' New Diet Revolution*, *The Carbohydrate Addict's Diet*, *Protein Power*, *Eat Fat, Get Thin* and *Diet Cure* were all appraised. None is recommended for weight loss and all could cause health problems.

No diet based on an excess of one constituent or a shortage of another will work long-term. I'm sorry to be boring but there is only one way to lose weight.

Chapter Eight
Losing It: The Bad News

If you have decided that weight loss is your only option, if you cannot accept yourself at the weight you are then, like me, you will want to ensure that this is the last time you ever diet.

So can you lose weight and keep it off permanently? Yes – it is possible. Very rare but certainly possible. What, you might ask cynically, can I suggest that will be different from what you and millions of others have done before, many times over, thus proving it doesn't work? What about the familiar recidivism figure: 95 per cent of weight lost is regained?

Well, here's the bad news. Weight loss is very, very tough. Don't believe anyone who tells you that they are on a plan on which they can eat so much that it doesn't feel like a diet. I've followed one of those plans for two and a half years and, although I believe it to be the best method going, I am still deprived. If it doesn't feel like a diet, the body won't be called upon to cannibalise itself.

This is not to say that losing weight means you have to go hungry. One of the main reasons for the failure of diets is that most of them are too low in calories to be sustained. You need not go hungry, though it is *normal* to experience some feelings of hunger.

Denial and Deprivation

Any weight-loss regime is divided into Can Have and Can't Have. The way this is done now is different from the bad old days when there were uncompromising lists of Foods You Can Eat Freely (lettuce, broccoli, green beans, tomatoes, white fish, grapefruit, cucumber, parsley, dandelion leaves), Foods You Can Eat Sparingly (meat, some fish, some fruit, small amounts of low-calorie cereal) and Foods You Touch on Pain of Death (bread, cheese, potatoes, sauce of any kind except vinegar, puddings, lots of fruits – like grapes – chocolate, alcohol . . . and anything else you might actually enjoy). These lists turned up in magazines, diet books and the diet sheets the GP used to give out when you went to him, cringing, because you felt you were too fat. The start of a diet was like hearing a prison gate clanging behind you, as you renounced the gustatory pleasures of the flesh. The emphasis, pre-1970s, was on low-carbohydrate regimes, so bread and potatoes were seen as twin evils (the only pasta we had then was macaroni). There was so much that you Couldn't Have that the diet was invariably abandoned in despair, and warmth, ecstasy and guilt flooded through you as you ravenously gobbled a hearty helping of Mum's meat pie with melt-in-the-mouth pastry and rich gravy.

Things are better ordered now. Most *balanced* diet regimes recognise that to ban a food is to make the dieter immediately crave it. Weight-loss plans tend to incorporate 'treats', even chocolate; the rationale is that a little of what you fancy not only does you good, it will enable you to stick to the diet. This makes a lot of sense – but you cannot eat freely. Whether you count calories, or use one of the slimming club methods of points or sins, there is a limit. There has to be. If it were not so, weight loss would be easy, the diet industry would be out of business and those carping fascists who nag on and on about the cost of obesity to the nation would have to go and look for another hapless group in society to target.

So you build the treat into your day – but you have to cut back on other things in order to incorporate it. You can't have the cake that someone has bought for the office to celebrate their birthday – or at least, not without a lot of borrowing and calculating and robbing Peter (tomorrow's allowance) to pay Paul (the extra you'll be consuming today). You can't sit down to a meal of lasagne, with fresh delicious wholemeal bread and real butter, followed by a pudding – well, you can, but you'll pay, either by going without 'treats' for a good few days or accepting that this week you won't lose weight. Or perhaps you won't eat anything else that day and end up with blood sugar so low that you fall over.

You do have to watch other people eating chocolate and cake and sandwiches and cheese and biscuits; you have to choose the lowest-calorie, lowest-fat option in a restaurant while your companion has leek and Brie pie followed by trifle. You have to watch as your family or friends grow mellow through the consumption of good wine while you remain clear-headed and sober after the one glass you've allowed yourself. While it's important to eat food you will enjoy, you can't eat just because food is enjoyable. You can't decide to have something because it looks or smells delicious, or because you just *feel* like it. Losing weight divests you of much of your free will. You can't indulge in *ad hoc* eating behaviour. My body sometimes feels like a battleground for my desire to eat like everyone else: just because it's *nice*.

Jill Welbourne, the eating disorders specialist, feels very strongly that dieters should not deprive themselves in the sense of refusing what it is they would most like to eat.

Say 'I'll just have one.' If you have one mince pie or whatever when you're first offered one, you avoid that feeling of deprivation. It takes away the power of the food. If you deprive yourself you'll end up eating the lot. I always tell people to hypnotise themselves by imagining the sound of a huge gong – like the J Arthur Rank gong at the beginning of films. Just hear it sounding a deep, resonant 'one'.

This can work but, again, only if you count carefully. That mince pie is at least 300 calories, about a fifth of the average daily allowance for someone of moderate overweight who is taking moderate exercise and trying to lose weight. For some it doesn't work because one helping of certain foods can trigger a binge. One mince pie may not feel enough when others are on their second. It can be easier to go without but this is a very individual thing. I would rather have no chocolate at all than a small piece which only stimulates my appetite for it and makes me long for more. I feel confident that I *can* manage small helpings of those 'trigger' foods; I'd just rather not have them. There is no doubt about the addictive qualities of certain types of food and, while a slim woman can afford a premenstrual chocolate binge once a month, a dieting woman cannot.

But it is not just those foods that the dieter misses. The things I feel deprived of are: fruit juice, nuts, seeds, chunks of wholemeal bread, muesli, olive oil, home-made pesto, dried fruit, peanut butter, apricot crumble, spinach quiche, roasted red pepper and goats cheese tart, the broccoli and Stilton pie that my local health food restaurant makes, and cheese. Cheddar cheese, sliced and eaten on a piece of toast spread with Marmite. Oh, and Parmesan. And things to drink that aren't no-cal. Of course I eat some of these things in small quantities. Occasionally. But it is not the same as being able to eat them freely or frequently.

I can't get away with normal eating: I've tried. If I go on holiday I eat 'normal' meals. I don't have puddings or ice creams. I drink Diet Coke, even though I worry about the chemicals in it. I don't eat between meals. And I invariably put on between 4 and 10 pounds.

Admittedly, some of the pounds are due to an increase in carbohydrate. No chemical processes can take place in the body unless the substances are in solution. When carbohydrate is digested it breaks down into a larger number of small molecules than fat or protein. Each molecule requires its own capsule of water so you gain weight by retaining fluid. Binge-eaters and bulimics can very quickly gain 5 lbs of which only 1 lb is tissue and the rest is fluid. The upside of this kind of gain is that the weight is usually lost fairly quickly, not by drastically reducing intake but by returning to the diet.

Deprivation and denial intrude on social eating too. Food is all around us; sharing it together is an essential part of the fabric of social life. 'Sharing food is love,' said the chef Ken Hom. I had expressed concern that he was standing alone in the kitchen doing all the work while the rest of us sat indolently around chatting. Most women are familiar with that sense of being excluded while they slave in the kitchen and their family or guests just enjoy themselves. But Ken saw it in a completely different way. For him, the creation of a beautiful meal is a way of expressing love and friendship. Sitting together and eating that meal is simply the next stage of a very important process.

One of my greatest deprivations (and I seem to come upon a lot of these) is the stand-up buffet. I love that food! Little sandwiches, sausage rolls, vol-au-vents, parcels of this and that, dips, flapjacks. My daughter's graduation, an aunt's ninetieth birthday, a party at a local drugs rehabilitation centre, the anniversary Mass of a friend's death – all recent occasions when people came together to celebrate, to mark an occasion, to share. If I'm invited to supper with friends I don't mention the diet; that would be to deny and defy the point of eating together. But I have to adjust my intake the next day.

Recently, I had lunch with a friend. It was a modest meal: a bit of ham, a little bread, a small salad and a piece of fruit afterwards. By about 5.30 p.m. we were peckish. She got out a packet of scones,

a pot of jam and a carton of cream. I had one scone – 200 calories.
My friend had two scones with jam and a lot of cream. If I had
eaten as she did I would have put on weight. She did not. This is
not due to different caloric expenditure – she's not keen on
exercise. It is because I have a dieted body and she does not. And it
will always be like this.

Barry Groves, author of several books on weight loss, says that
he and his wife had a problem with overweight. They had tried all
the usual reduction methods to no avail. Then walking through a
Singapore market they came upon a book which advocated an
unrestricted calorie diet for weight loss. In as many words this book
said: eat as many calories as you like and the pounds will fall off.
Groves and his wife thought they had nothing to lose (as it were)
by trying this method and decided to see what it could do for them.
He says it worked and has worked for over thirty-seven years.[1]

What a dream! All I can say is that the times in my life when I
have gained weight are those when I have eaten unrestricted
calories. Maybe the Groves have a different metabolic make-up or
genetic profile from the rest of us. I can only say that their method
does not work for me, more's the pity.

There are two ways of viewing this denial and deprivation
business. You can say 'My diet is great: I can have a glass of wine*
with a meal.' Modern weight-loss methods certainly do allow this
luxury (it's only a question of allocation of calories, nothing
magical). Or you can view the glass as half-empty – almost literally!
In which case you will say 'I can only have one glass of wine on this
lousy diet; what kind of life is that?'

A Life Sentence

Whichever method you choose to lose weight, this will be the way
you will have to live for the rest of your life. If you have become

---

*Or six rich tea biscuits at bedtime – the dubious treat of a friend of mine
– or any other little calorific extravagance that tickles your tastebuds. If I
put this weight back on it will be because I've fallen prey to the siren song
of dried fruit. I record this now so that if it happens, and my critics say
that I've obviously started stuffing myself with doughnuts, you can write
in and say 'She didn't, M'Lud. It was the dried figs what did for her.'

overweight by eating thousands of 'empty' calories – that is, by filling yourself with processed high-fat, high-sugar foods – the change of regimen should not be too onerous, though I fear that the simple switch from 'bad' to 'good' foods will not be all it takes for most people to reduce their weight significantly.

Some people claim they lose weight when they stop dieting. I am always slightly cynical about this: it sounds too good to be true and if it were that easy, we would all do it (another way to confound the obesity fascists). But what do people mean when they say this? I think what happens is that they have been used to living on an exhausting see-saw of low-calorie diets with typical dieter's mentality. They start fad, or low-calorie diets, one after the other. They lose weight, they come off the diet, they regain the weight plus more, they hear about a new diet and try that – and so the yo-yo keeps swinging. By this time, they have reached an all-time high weight. Then they see the light, realise that these diets don't work and start eating properly, perhaps for the first time in years. Their weight stabilises; they may even lose a little.

If, after this, people do actually return from a high to an average weight without trying, they are the lucky ones who can reduce their calorie intake virtually without effort. But if they lose weight, they must be eating less than their body needs, otherwise it would not be cannibalising itself.

Most people are not so lucky. As you can see from the calorie requirement chart in the Appendix, it works like this: the heavier you are, the more you can eat. A heavy body requires more calories just to keep it going. And it uses up more calories with every movement it makes. If your daily intake consists of say, 3000 calories, and you are a high but stable weight, you will start to lose by reducing to 2500 and moving around a little more. You will still be eating a very generous amount of food and you won't feel as though you are dieting. For instance, if you are aged between 18 and 29, weigh 17 stone and lead a pretty sedentary life your calorie requirement will be 3130 a day. If you cut that by 500, you will lose about a pound a week and still be eating over 2500 calories per day. If you take some exercise your calorie requirement at that weight goes up to 3548. Although that would mean you would lose weight a little faster because of the extra calories expended in exercise, it would be advisable to eat a little more and stick to the pound a week loss.

While the calorie requirement chart is a useful way of determining how much you can eat to lose, or maintain, weight, you need to take into account your own individual metabolism. The dieted body functions more efficiently than the non-dieted one in its ability to conserve the calories you eat; it is not such a spendthrift. This is even more true of the much-dieted body.

'Yo-yo dieters have tuned their metabolism to be super-efficient,' says Jill Welbourne. 'Fourteen or fifteen years of yo-yo dieting with no intervening stable period will make one calorie do what two did previously.'

So, in order to find out how much you can safely eat, start from the figure given in the Basal Metabolic Rate (BMR) column. As this is calculated on a 'lying in a coma' state, it will allow for any reduction in metabolic rate brought about by dieting. And you may well be able to eat more than this, especially if you are active. You should not need to eat less than your BMR figure.

But as your weight decreases, so does your body's basic calorie requirement. Your lighter body does not need as much fuel to keep it going, so in order to carry on losing weight your calorie intake has to go down (or your energy output go up). This is the booby prize of weight loss: the more you lose, the less you can eat. You do your body a favour by taking the strain off its poor joints and it rewards you by saying 'Thanks. That's much better. But I'm not a Rolls-Royce any more, I'm a Ford now so I don't need as much fuel.' So when you get down to, say, 13 stone, (aged 18–29) your sedentary calorie requirement is 2640 and your active requirement, 2990.

Unfortunately, daily calorie requirements lessen with age. So the 17-stone woman aged 30–59 needs 2584 (sedentary) and 2929 (active). The 13-stone woman of that age requires 2300 (sedentary) or 2600 (active).

The calorie-requirement table differs from the BMI chart in that its figures are provable. It is not subjective; science can measure how many calories you use. The BMI chart, with its bands of normal, overweight, obese and morbidly obese, immediately labels you. And there is *still* no universal agreement about the health risks pertaining to each band.

Besides, since researching this book, I have discovered any variations of the BMI chart. Superficially, they look the same with their vertical banding and shading, but my own degree of overweight seems to vary with each one. Hardly scientifically consistent.

Not only does less flesh mean less energy (calories) required, but the efficient body slows down your metabolic rate when you lose weight. Don't forget, your body has a mind of its own. When it has to burn its own fat stores as fuel it has only one response: it thinks there is a famine. Your body is your friend, it wants to keep you alive. It will hold on to as much of itself as it can so that it can keep going for the maximum amount of time, with any luck until the season of famine passes. It also wants to hang on to its insulation – like the lagging on a hot-water tank – in case famine brings hypothermia with it.

The majority of obesity experts, most of whom have never carried an ounce of surplus flesh, claim that when you stop dieting your metabolic rate returns to normal. I don't believe the so-called experts. They do not take the individual into account. They measure everything in calorimeter chambers; they don't look at real-life situations or the fluctuations in body rhythms. They certainly don't seem to take your psychology into account, nor the fact that you can eat fewer calories as the weight drops, nor that your body defends its weight. They insist that everyone's metabolic rate is the same and that thin people always eat less than fat ones.

Because these experts work on cold facts and statistics, they have no idea what it is like to live with a high body weight; they have little notion about what repeated dieting does to the mind and the spirit; and they do not know first hand what happens when you have lost weight. Their interpretation of overeating does not take into account emotional eating nor the desperate need to eat that comes from too many incidences of near starvation on low-calorie diets. In fact, many of them, completely ignoring the life-long problems that these diets can set in motion, still recommend low-calorie diets. And when people fail on them, because no one can spend their life on a low-calorie diet, the pundits pass sentence: early death for fat sinners. They are like the righteous thin in a medieval painting: on their way straight to heaven, while the fat are herded off to hell. There is the same judgemental cast about them.

So what you hear, on the subject of recidivism, is that people have 'gone back to their bad old ways' (or as Vanessa Feltz would have it, to 'shoving doughnuts down their cakehole');[2] that it isn't the diet that's failed, it's the dieter. Not true. What usually happens is that people finish the diet, feel good about their achievement and then return to *normal* eating. You can't do it. Your body will be fighting to regain the weight you have lost and more.

This can be clearly seen in the typical pattern of weight loss. Although I have lost six and a half stone, the first two went fairly easily, the second two required a lot more effort and the last two stone took ages. In fact, it took a whole year to lose the final stone. My body had marshalled its defences against this unnatural thing I was doing to it. Originally, I had planned to lose about eight stone but this was not to be. Jill Welbourne explained why my weight loss had stopped.

> You have lost six stone over several years so your body believes you are in a country where there is a chronic sub-famine. The body knows that it has had to reduce its tissues; that you are in a state of tissue loss. Three quarters of a pound a week puts it into conserve mode – that's why you are cold.

Just to prove further its considerable survival skills, the dieted body sends a signal to what I think of as the 'housekeeping' enzyme: lipoprotein lipase. The job of this bustling little chemical is to help deposit fat in your fat cells, even though you don't want it to, thank you very much. When you lose large amounts of weight this enzyme gets a move on. As soon as you try to return to anything approaching 'normal' eating, it becomes extremely busy, squirrelling away fat at a much faster rate than normal. It is rather like those very annoying people who start panic buying at the whisper of a shortage: you know, they'll buy sixteen loaves of bread and shove them in the freezer. Lipoprotein lipase does the same, only with fat.

If you need any more convincing about your body's superefficient ability to regain its lost weight, then just envisage this. Every time we get larger, more adipocytes (fat cells) are created to hold the extra fat. When weight is lost, a large number of these adipocytes reluctantly release their contents. But these cells don't disappear, they hang around redundantly like empty grain stores waiting for the harvest to come in. When it does, the body celebrates.

The unpalatable fact, the truth that is shunned by dieters and anti-diet activists alike, is that if you lose weight you will have to stay on a diet for life. As Jill Welbourne puts it succinctly: 'You can never go back because losing weight means that what was once a weight-maintaining diet becomes a weight-gaining diet.'

Even a slow loss, say a pound a week, sets off the famine alarm. In other words, you can never eat normally again. Do you hear the clang of the prison door slamming shut?

Set Point Theory and Why You Have to Exercise the Dreaded Dietary Discipline

This means that your body has a self-determined weight at which it is healthy and comfortable. This may be nothing like that of the useless height/weight tables and it may not put you into the 'normal' section of the BMI chart either. No matter. If you eat healthily and exercise moderately, with no thought of body size or dieting (faint hope), you will be the weight you were meant to be, whether this is 7 stone or 13. You will not have to 'watch your weight', you can enjoy food and never count a calorie.

There is a great deal of controversy and argument about set point theory, though all the common-sense research I have read suggests incontrovertibly that set point exists. If the set point theory were more widely accepted and the model adapted to the practice of modern medicine we would see a decline in the pursuit of the 'ideal' body size because people would have a better understanding of individuality. Just as hair texture differs from fine and wispy to thick and heavy, so set point defines your own genetically determined body size. If you are meant to be 5' 5" and 12^1/$_2$ stone, there is no point in dieting to be 8^1/$_2$.

Pre-determined genetic set point is one thing: I am convinced that my own natural body weight is around 11 stone. But repeated weight loss and regain raises the set point each time, so that your 'natural' body weight becomes higher and higher. You have convinced your body that it has to maintain a high weight because it is under threat. The image of the fat person screaming to get out of the thin(ner) body bears some relation to the truth if you are using food restriction to maintain a lower weight than

is natural for you, or if you have lost weight and regained it
several times.

Here's an example. My friend Maggie was a slim, glamorous,
blonde television presenter in the 1970s. Her weight was stable
at 10 stone and she ate anything and everything she wanted. She
had a particular fondness for fried eggs! In the late eighties, after
her TV career, she weighed 11 st 2 lbs, an ideal weight for her
height of 5′ 8″ and a normal, middle-aged increase, but Maggie
did not like being that big – she felt it wasn't 'her'. She
embarked on several sessions of the Cambridge Diet, a VLCD
that allowed her less than 500 calories a day. She lost some
weight – not a lot, but enough to make her feel more
'acceptable'. It was hard going and she didn't feel good: her
diary records that she was 'feeling rather light-headed. Had to
stop weeding.' She also *gained* weight during some phases of this
starvation diet.

In Maggie's words the Cambridge Diet 'buggered up' her
metabolism completely. After it, she steadily gained until she
was 13 stone. Her set point, knowing what was good for her and
what definitely wasn't, had adjusted itself to a higher setting,
leaving her heavier than she had ever been or wanted to be.

In May 2000, hoping to lull her body into believing it wasn't
dieting, Maggie began a sensible reducing plan based on the
body's diurnal rhythms, eating a normal breakfast and lunch
with just vegetables for supper. By doing this she cut her calories
very gradually and lost 19 lbs in 10 months. The weight loss
plateaued at that point but Maggie was much happier with
herself and remained a steady 11 stone 9 lbs.

Then she got a taste for Eccles cakes, and why not? She didn't
binge or go mad. Still maintaining her body clock eating plan,
Maggie ate 20 Eccles cakes in a month – less than one per day.
She is physically active. In that month she put on 5 lbs. Now, even
the most purist of obesity pundits, the most fanatical weight
fascist, could not accuse Maggie of overeating by having less than
one Eccles cake a day. But once you've dieted, you can't do it.

It is because of the inconveniently self-adjusting set point that
you can never relax. You will have to observe what one prissy
(thin of course) obesity 'expert' refers to as Dietary Discipline
and maintain it for ever and ever. Amen.

The Trivialisation of Weight Loss

I have no patience with vanity dieters: the women who want to lose weight to look good in a bikini; the perfectly normal weight ones who would like to be 'just half a stone lighter'; the size 12s who yearn to be size 10. I don't care that the majority of 'normal' weight women are insecure about their bodies; I am unmoved by their plight.

The reason for this hard-heartedness is twofold. Firstly, I despair at a society which has become so affluent that it is reduced to focusing with such intense attention on matters that are purely cosmetic. Where food is plentiful, where consumerism and materialism have replaced religion and spirituality, there are deep levels of dissatisfaction and often the only focus for this is a trivial one. Thus people set great store by appearances of all kinds and intelligence, ability, humour and personality are subjugated to the cult of The Look.

The feminist writer, Suzanne Moore, in a piece about death from anorexia, observed that even the most extreme of circumstances – when women die from self-induced starvation – do not lead other women to question their obsession with thinness:

> We worry about models being too skinny and girls as young as seven saying that they are too fat but ask most women what it is that they want, they really, really want and they will tell you that their lives would be entirely different if they lost half a stone. Bridget Jones's obsession with her calorie intake makes us laugh precisely because we identify with it even as we recognise its silliness.[3]

Secondly, writing and broadcasting about the subject for nearly twenty years has brought me into contact with hundreds of women who have suffered unbearably from the slings and arrows of outrageous misfortune; from the abuse, persecution, prejudice and discrimination hurled at them because of their size. Women who are only a couple of stone 'overweight' are made to feel sinners. It can be particularly hard for young women who feel ostracised because they are a size 14 or 16 and therefore ineligible for the 'cool gang'.

I am tired and bored with a lifetime of dietspeak amongst women. When women get together the conversation nearly always turns to weight. Whatever feminism has achieved, it has not managed to liberate women from the narcissistic obsession with the way they look. Nor has it made them more charitable about the way other women look. It is just one big competition. I belong to a group of highly successful, extremely intelligent women writers. We meet once a month for a whole day during which we work hard and break to have lunch together. There is a dreadful, predictable ritualistic component to these days: the commenting on weight which appears to be as essential as 'Hello, how are you?'

It goes like this. The women arrive and we have a cup of tea or coffee before we start work. As we see each other only once a month, catching up on news is embarked upon. This is peppered with weight-related remarks. 'A, you're looking very slender, have you lost weight?' A replies that she has not, in fact she may even have put some weight on. Then someone will comment that B is looking 'marvellous' – she's lost weight. As far as I can see, the members of the group have remained around the same size since we began meeting many years ago, but the ritual dance has to take place before the real work can be done.

Ironically, only one member of the group – the one who doesn't join in this boring exchange – has commented on my weight loss, and she did so privately.

Fat people rarely join in conversations about weight. It is too painful. With rare exceptions it is only if women are quite confident that they could not in any *objective* sense be called fat that they are able to talk about the subject with other people.

So Should You Try to Lose Weight?

Some people cannot lose weight because it would harm their psychological health if they tried to live with the deprivation that even a moderate dieting regime brings with it. When people are trying to cope with large amounts of pressure, with life events that register in the top five of the most stressful things that can befall you, or when they are clinically depressed, losing weight would only add to the load they are already bearing.

There is only one good reason for embarking on a weight-loss programme and that is that you are certain that you have no alternative: that for physical and/or psychological reasons you cannot go on existing in your overweight body.

Being fat is painful. It puts you out in the cold; you belong only by virtue of being able to offer compensations for your size. If you are funny, sympathetic, outrageous, you may be able to make your mark. If you do not have something else to offer then you feel isolated.

I understand so well what it feels like to know that, whatever your political beliefs, you yourself would live a happier, fuller and healthier life if you were less fat. It is that which is the only reason for losing weight: your own well-being.

But I believe you should set yourself conditions. First, you need to be absolutely confident in your ability to lose weight and keep it off permanently. This may mean sorting out your eating before you begin: identifying the reasons why you became fat in the first place; being completely honest about the role food has played in your life; understanding what your relationship with food is about. If you do not know these things you will come a cropper. You will just repeat all those other attempts to lose weight when it has all returned to you with interest.

You also need a period of psychological preparation. During this time you should think about what weight loss will mean: the deprivation, the denial, the discipline (all the unpleasant Ds!). You need to look ahead, not months or even years, but to the end of your life. What you are contemplating is for ever. There is never any going back if the loss is to be permanent.

You have to be absolutely wholehearted. You even need to be a bit obsessional (though it's not a good thing to bore others with your new eating plan or your weight loss!). You have to keep very focused because you will be doing something that is not natural and it is easy to lose sight after while. You may become blasé and complacent, especially after a couple of stone have gone, but if you do you'll find yourself gaining half a stone before you know it. *You* may think you're doing your body a favour; *it* wants to retain the status quo.

Planning the diet is important, as in evaluating the different methods: slimming club, counting calories, points, sins, exercise. Consider where your support will be coming from. Give yourself time, before you start, to work out what you really want to do.

It took me two years to decide to diet for the last time. I was actually very scared of the idea. Scared of giving up the food I loved, of not having enough to eat, of failing. Scared most of all of losing weight and putting it back on again.

I firmly believe that the decision to lose weight has to be like the decision to get married or have a baby. It is not something you should drift into – at least that's the way I feel about marriage and babies; you may not. And I am not saying that deciding to lose weight has the same life importance as those other two events! But the feeling of certainty must be the same, the feeling that now is the right time for the right reasons.

There is a moment when you know, without a doubt, that you want to lose weight. It's like a switch being thrown; you recognise it straightaway when it happens. I waited for that moment for two years and I cannot define the difference between my thinking time and the moment I made the decision. I do know that if I had started my diet during the first period it would have failed. I had to reach that point of complete readiness.

Don't underestimate the importance and commitment of this decision. Casual dieting is bad for anyone, both physically and psychologically. But it is particularly bad for the very large person who has known disappointment and defeat many times before. Someone like that, like me, cannot afford to put weight on again.

This diet, unlike the others, does not have an end. So the only good reason for undertaking it is that you want to lose weight so badly you are prepared to work at it for life.

A Diet by Any Other Name...

'We don't like to call this a diet, we like to call it a healthy-eating plan.' This was said to me by representatives of slimming organisations and authors of diet books. The euphemisms still prevail. As I hope I have made clear, I think diet is the only word to use. If you've made the decision to lose weight, you will have to diet.

The trouble is that *diets*, in the way the twentieth century came to understand them, involved adopting an idiosyncratic, exotic, non-nutritious or just plain impossible way of eating. You could do it but you could only do it for a finite amount of time. Diets, by definition, were something you went on and came off. They started on a Monday and were more often than not abandoned by Friday. There was no way you could make them a permanent way of life. When I was eating two grapefruit for lunch every single day during the year I dieted for my wedding, it did not occur to me that I would not be able to keep that up for ever. I'd fallen into the trap of following a goal-oriented diet. I reached the goal, thankfully dropped the diet and put on four stone in two years.

Like Jill Welbourne, I do not altogether like the word 'diet' because it implies something temporary. But I cannot entirely agree with her alternative: permanent, pleasant lifestyle changes. The essence of that is undoubtedly true but the word 'pleasant' makes it an intrinsically flawed definition; it contains assumptions. While this is subjective to some degree, the hard fact is that losing weight entails deprivation and some people cannot bear that.

Lifestyle changes *are* important and they do need to be permanent. If you are eating high-fat food, junk food and not enough fruit or vegetables or complex carbohydrates, then you need to change the way you eat – for ever. If you sit around like a slug all day (and some days I do – it's difficult for a writer with deadlines not to), you've got to get your body moving. The quality of what you eat and of how you treat your body is as important as the dieting part of weight loss.

As for weight loss through exercise – well, perhaps it's time someone wrote a book called *Exercise Makes You Fat*. Huge amounts of vigorous exercise – the type you get in a long, hard workout at the gym, something that takes perhaps two to three hours – will cause you to lose vast quantities of weight very quickly, especially if you cut down your food intake and eat low-fat foods. The results can be quite magical. But can you really go to the gym in this way for the rest of your life? If you think you can, fine. If you are going to be a sixty-year-old Jane Fonda type, good luck to you. But most people won't stick it. And because the weight loss has depended on frequent, hard exercise, as soon as you let go – even just a little – the weight will hasten gleefully back to resettle all over you, bringing some more with it as insurance against the same thing happening again.

As long as you realise you are going to have to diet, it doesn't matter what you personally choose to call it. There are any number of ways you can achieve weight loss but whichever way you go about it, the fact is that you must become a cannibal and feed off your own body.

The body doesn't know it is too fat. What it does know is that it has to hang on to its fat stores, especially if it's had the sniff of a famine around. Once you have dieted, you will always have a tendency to put on weight. Reaching a stable weight and staying there means that you have got the energy balance right. Tiny adjustments in intake and output will make a difference but it will be very, very slow. I know of a woman who lost 15 lbs by doing nothing but give up her evening glass of sherry. It took about a year, though. For most large people, embarking on a diet – and this is the last ever one, remember – is a scary prospect. But it is also an exciting one as long as you are prepared to be patient.

And I am suggesting you lose weight very, very slowly. No other way will work in the long term. My six and a half stone weight loss worked out at an average of three quarters of a pound a week. About three pounds a month. It was fast enough. But as a 'Diet', it would not have a scrap of commercial potential!

In Summary

- Losing weight is tough
- You will experience denial and deprivation
- You will have to practise Dietary Discipline and you will want to rebel
- You will never be able to eat normally again if you want to keep the weight off
- Your metabolic rate drops
- Your body defends its set point weight and will fight to regain it
- If you are helping your weight loss with exercise, you will have to keep that up for life, too – or reduce your calorie intake further
- The more weight you lose, the less you can eat – the booby prize
- You will need to remain constantly vigilant
- You may never reach your desired weight. At 13 stone I am still in the upper limits of 'overweight' on the BMI chart. I am still seen as a fat woman

In Conclusion

I have given you the bad news. Since this is not a diet book, I have told the truth. Any diet book that came clean about the arduous task of weight loss and weight maintenance would not sell many copies. They all promise easy solutions. There aren't any.

The good news, from one who has been there, is that the benefits far outweigh the difficulties. I love being thinner. I have greater confidence and higher self-esteem. I wish that it did not have to take weight loss to do that for me, but I have to deal in my reality as it is and not as I would like it to be. I never achieved a sense of harmony or wholeness with my very large body though I tried very hard indeed to accept it. It was a little like an atheist trying to believe in God: no matter how many believers try to convince you, or to persuade you to join them, if it doesn't ring true in your own heart, it cannot happen.

Jill Welbourne once said to me that there were no health risks in being overweight until you got to the point where you couldn't tie your own shoelaces. I didn't wear shoes with laces but I was uncomfortably aware that this was probably just as well since tying them every day would have presented a bit of a challenge. I was too heavy, too big, not by anyone else's definition but my own. I did not care about conforming to the social or medical parameters of what size was acceptable: where they are concerned I am still not an acceptable size but that's fine by me.

I would never have weight-loss surgery. I do not believe in the concept or the practice of eating abnormally small amounts of food, nor of having my body mutilated. Neither would I take weight-loss drugs. They are still an unknown quantity. Besides, the joke about these drugs is that they have to be accompanied by a reduction in calories. All those risks and you still have to diet.

I had lived for years with the belief that permanent weight loss was an impossible goal because so few achieved it. I'd failed to achieve it myself, many times. Whenever I thought about having another try, all I could think of was that recidivism figure: 95 per cent.

What changed my mind was a blinding flash of the bleeding obvious. I turned that figure on its head. If that percentage of weight losers put it all on again – *what about the 5 per cent who keep it off* ? Why should I not be in that part of the statistic? Once you start thinking like that, your motivation comes from an entirely different place: a positive place.

For many, life will be too short to diminish its quality by dieting. For others, life is too short not to.

Chapter Nine
How to Lose Weight (and Keep Your Sanity)

There is no point in trying to lose weight unless you are prepared to be patient and lose it slowly. You cannot lose more than a kilo (2.2 lbs) of fat in a week no matter what diet you follow. Any weight loss greater than that will be fluid or muscle mass. Not only is this highly dangerous but when you regain the weight (and you will for certain if you lose it fast) you'll put back fat instead of muscle. You'll be physically messed up, you'll feel a failure and you won't have done your health any good.

Ideally, you should eat so that you lose an average of half a pound a week to give you the best chance of keeping the weight off. That may sound unbearably tedious and unrewarding but it will result in a loss of two stone in a year. If you really can't bear that, go for a pound but you'll probably find that after a year or so it will slow down anyway. Even with a very slow weight loss the body is like a particularly vigilant watchdog, nose in the air for the smell of food shortages. Even though I am no longer losing, my body is on famine alert all the time. Ideally, I should have been content with half a pound a week but I had a great deal of weight to lose and I don't have age on my side.

Okay, so you're going to do it – but only if you are utterly convinced that this will be the last time in your life that you lose weight. The diet, or 'eating plan', must be one that suits you and later on I will give details of some of the better ones. But there is no magic in this. You have to change your energy balance. I used to think it was far more complicated than that, and indeed it can be where food is serving an important psychological purpose. That is a subject all of its own. But I've been doing it for nearly three years and I have lost weight; although I've felt deprived, I've never actually felt starved, weak or ill. On previous diets I had felt all of those things and no one can live like that unless they are in a country or situation where there is absolutely no choice. The cost is too high; the health consequences are too risky and the goal – permanent weight loss – is unattainable.

First some facts about weight loss.

What You Should Know About Calories

There are 3500 calories in a pound of fat. In order to put on one pound you have to consume 3500 calories *more* than your body needs. This is rather hard to believe as any woman knows how quickly she can put on several pounds without having been on an eating bender, but that's the chemistry of it. One explanation for weight gain is that there are all sorts of circumstances that contribute to fluid retention but, for actual fat to be laid down, you must ingest 3500 spare calories for every pound.

If, though, you are not what Jill Welbourne calls an 'unmodified human being' (in other words, if you have been a serial dieter), your over-efficient body will see to it that you put on a pound of fat long before you've eaten that 3500-calorie excess.

And incidentally, this whole business of putting on weight is about more than gaining fat and fluid. When you get bigger, your body has to manufacture more blood vessels and more blood, to serve the extra tissue being laid down. Your bone density increases too, which is one of the reasons why large women are rarely at risk of osteoporosis.

If you eat 100 calories a day more than your body needs you will gain 10 pounds a year. If you eat 100 calories less, you'll lose 10 pounds in a year. So cutting your daily intake by 500 calories will result in a loss of about a pound a week.

But a reduction of 500 calories can feel quite drastic, though it depends on how many you were eating before you started the diet. If it was 3000 then 2500 won't seem too bad, but it's all relative. If you increase your output by 250 calories, say, you can cut intake by only 250. The secret of successful weight loss is to create a fine, careful balance between intake and expenditure so that you eat enough to be able to stick to it, exercise enough to burn off calories that otherwise would turn to fat and do the whole thing very slowly so that the changes you make are as minimal as possible to get a long-term result.

Simplifying Metabolism

Metabolic rate are two words much bandied about where weight loss is concerned and the phrase is understood by many to mean the basic mechanism for fatness, thinness and weight changes.

While this is part of it, metabolism is rather more complicated than just the process that makes you gain or lose weight.

Metabolism is the sum total of all the chemical reactions taking place in your body at any one time. There are two sorts of reactions: anabolic and catabolic. Anabolic reactions build you up (as in anabolic steroids); catabolic reactions break you down. Anabolic processes are to do with growth, development, the formation of bone, muscle and tissue, healing and repairing. Catabolic processes are at play during illness, exhaustion and weight loss. The sum total of all these processes is the metabolic rate. The balance between them is called homeostasis.

The metabolism is like a fire: it requires fuel in order to work. If fuel is short, the fire burns more slowly and the heat diminishes. If you are short of food, ie on a calorie-restricted diet, all the processes in your body slow down so that you can conserve as much as possible of what is coming in. Your temperature and your blood pressure will fall (the latter may make you feel a bit dizzy) and your heart rate will be slower.

Jill Welbourne likens this shortage to someone being on a restricted or reduced income. Because there is less money coming in you save on non-essential items. You turn off the radiators in the bedroom and hall and just leave one on in the main living room. You cut down on phone calls, buy cheaper food, mend clothes – anything to save enough to keep the vital, core processes going. And that is a reduced metabolic rate – there is less going on. Your body will housekeep in the same way, making cuts wherever possible. This is why your metabolic rate falls when you go on a diet, any diet. You are in negative energy balance. Normal energy balance exists when calorie intake and output are equal and weight stays stable. Positive energy balance occurs when we take in more calories than the body expends.

Energy in this respect has three components:

The resting metabolic rate. This is the amount of energy you burn doing absolutely nothing and that would be burned if you were lying in a coma. This accounts for 60–70 per cent of calories used.

Thermogenesis. Energy used to keep warm, digest food and respond to stress.

Physical activity. This includes all movement from raising your eyebrows to running a marathon. Included in this is non-exercise activity thermogenesis (NEAT). NEAT could be described as purposeless activity and includes fidgeting, twitching, constantly moving your body, even talking. The old idea that some people are thin because they use up so much nervous energy ('she's never still') has considerable accuracy. People under stress do tend to lose weight (unless they comfort eat to combat the stress) because they find it hard to relax and engage in a lot of twitchy, restless movement.

Jill Welbourne and some colleagues did a very interesting comparison of metabolic rates, looking at pairs of people in similar situations: a boss and his secretary; two people training (one of whom had a sedentary job) for different athletic events; a consultant and a junior doctor; and two old ladies in a home. They compared the difference in energy expenditure between each couple. The secretary's output was greater than her boss's: she had to run around more, including up and down stairs to the photocopier. The junior doctor cycled to work while the consultant took the car. But the biggest difference was between the two old ladies, apparently in the same situation. One of them sat in a chair most of the day, using a zimmer frame to walk. The other had dementia and her anxiety caused her to wander ceaselessly. Her expenditure was around 4000 calories a day and she got increasingly thinner because her food intake wasn't sufficient to match it. She was, in effect, on a perfect diet. Out of everyone studied, the old lady's energy output was by far the greatest.

The Role of Exercise in Weight Loss

Here's the good news then – you don't have to do aerobics to lose weight. You don't even have to do aerobic exercise for five thirty-minute periods a week, or twenty minutes twice a day or any of those other things usually recommended. If a wandering old lady can burn off 4000 calories, strictly unaerobically, there's hope for us all.

We've all heard about the old days, when we were all much more active, and it's true. We don't move enough now and we don't use up enough calories in exercise. If you're a mother, on the go all day, pushing a pram, doing housework, walking to school to fetch the children, you will be burning up huge amounts without – apparently – taking anything that most people nowadays would recognise as exercise (because most people are fixated on the gym or aerobics classes). If you're a keen gardener, walker or sports player, you'll be doing fine. But most of us now simply don't move our bodies around enough.

Using a table produced by the Calorie Control Council[1] I calculated my energy expenditure for a very active day (in my dreams!).

In this imaginary day, I got up and brushed my teeth for 5 minutes (17 cals). Then I did 30 minutes housework (263 cals) and 20 minutes ironing (62 cals). I walked to the supermarket, 15 mins there, 15 mins back (126 cals) and spent 30 minutes doing the shopping (148 cals). During the afternoon I did 10 minutes disco dancing (70 cals) and played the piano for 15 minutes (58 cals). After having friends for supper it took me 15 minutes to clear up (93 cals). During the course of the day I spent five minutes running up and down stairs (62 cals).

The activities I have listed burned 899 calories. They would only have formed a part of the energy I would have expended as I have not included *everything* I would do in an active day. Every movement uses up calories – even typing this book is energy expenditure. Just moving from room to room, washing up, brushing hair, opening a can of cat food: an endless list of small daily tasks all of which add to the total calories burned.

My resting metabolic rate is 1532; my body requires that number of calories to keep me alive without losing weight. If my intake on this particular day had been the recommended 2000 for women, then the difference between intake and output would have created an enormous calorie deficit (ie 431). If every day was like that I would lose weight pretty quickly.

It does begin to make you see why fatness is now so prevalent and why the wartime generation ate far more than we do today and yet weighed less. Doing that calculation has made me resolve to be more generally active. Modern living has made things too easy. We save a great number of calories by using the remote control for the television, for instance, and by typing on a computer keyboard instead of the old manual typewriters, which required far greater pressure and the use of muscles to swing back the carriage return after every line typed. Those are just two examples of the way technology and lifestyle changes have worked insidiously to curtail the amount we move our bodies.

So if you are to create the negative energy balance necessary for weight loss, it pays to burn calories in exercise that you can sustain daily. There are simple things you can do. It does not have to be a big production but it does have to be a way of life that can take in the effects of ageing and generally slowing down. It's no good taking up jogging every day before breakfast if you have to give it up later because your knees have gone, or you can't face early mornings any more.

Consistent, regular exercise also helps to keep the metabolic clock ticking over, helping to counteract the effects of the reduced metabolic rate caused by dieting.

You can try to alter the basics: little things like doing hand washing occasionally, not using the TV remote (getting up and down to adjust volume and switch the set on and off burns an astonishing number of calories!) and making yourself walk as much as possible, even if it's only from one room to another. Walk to work if possible, or cycle. Stairs are excellent; find reasons to run upstairs a number of times a day. Just keep moving – look for every opportunity, however small, to shift your body around. Remember – *all* movement burns calories.

For general fitness and weight loss you need to incorporate some sustained exercise into your life but it should be something that fits easily, not something you have to make an effort to go and do. If you join an exercise class or make a commitment to go swimming it will help but will you be able to keep it up? I'm positive that home-based exercise is the best. Walking is excellent and really cannot be bettered – if you enjoy it.

As for duration, recent research has shown that exercise bouts of only ten minutes, two or three times a day, can be very effective in losing weight. Glenn Gaesser, an exercise physiologist at the University of Virginia, reasoned that people just don't have time for the 30–60 minute periods of sustained aerobic exercise that are traditionally recommended. Gaesser discovered research which showed that three ten-minute bursts had the same benefits as one 30-minute workout.

He devised a programme for a sedentary group of 40 women consisting of 15 ten-minute bursts of exercise per week. In three weeks they lost weight, improved their fitness levels and had reduced levels of cholesterol and triglycerides. The results the women achieved would normally be expected to take three months with a traditional exercise programme. The reason for this startling result is that during and after exercise the body releases growth hormone, an important muscle-building and fat-mobilising chemical. Three daily surges of this hormone confer triple the benefits of one daily surge.[2]

No more working up a sweat or getting exhausted. Ten minutes short sharp exercise makes you feel good. I've tried it and recommend it. It's far less painless in every sense than my 35-minute hill slog.

In addition to walking, cycling, dancing or whatever form of exercise turns you on (and apparently exercise is very good for that, and 'that' is very good exercise!), isometrics are also efficient calorie burners. These are stationary exercises that use the large groups of muscles: they burn a lot of energy. So if you work sitting at a desk, clench your buttocks and let go, as many times in the day as you can remember to do so. Lean, or push hard, against a wall, pull your stomach and back in and hold it. Do the pelvic floor exercises.

And fidget. If you are deskbound – and I'm very conscious that a writer's life is extremely deskbound – tap your feet, sway from side to side, stop and swing your arms, rotate your ankles. Of course it's alright for me in the privacy of my own home – but do what you can! Using a keyboard is quite good, though not as good as the electric typewriter was and not half as good as the old manuals where you really had to thump and return a great heavy carriage every few seconds.

If you are very large you may feel anxious about taking exercise because it can be difficult. I am convinced that unless someone has a physical disability, reticence about exercising the large body springs from the assumptions of others that fat people can't. Can't move, can't run, can't dance: it's all part of the negative stereotype imposed on us. We don't have to buy it. Large bodies usually have an astonishing grace and rhythm; flesh flows in ways that bones cannot.

Dancing is great if you are large and belly dancing is superb. No one can belly dance as sensuously as a fat woman. Television producer Jane Goddard Carter used to be diffident about her large body until she realised that the best way to answer her detractors was to show them what she could do. She took up belly dancing:

> Now I boldly dance, leap, lift and astound. I endure. I have stamina and strength. I have agility and elegance. I have style – big dramatic hair, clothes, a rhythmic gait, expansive gestures. I shine, I really do. Whenever and wherever I can, I live it to the full. I use the shape of my body and the shape of my mind to be lively, sharp and sensuous... Yes, I do dance well, certainly not in spite of my size, but because of it. Belly dancing requires a belly and a good weighty arse. I have got both, nice ones, too! I love it when a shimmy takes on a life of its own: it looks and feels wonderful. Shock and surprise on the faces of others are rewards as well.[3]

Kathryn Szrodecki is a fitness instructor who runs aerobics classes for large women. Kathryn herself is very large and she is proof that a high level of fitness and a high weight are perfectly compatible. Because she understands what it is to be fat she has a gift for freeing large women from the confines of embarrassment about their bodies and from the conviction that their bodies will not perform for them in the way that thinner women's do. She exposes the mythology of this and her classes demonstrate her philosophy, with large women bending and stretching and moving and dancing in joyful liberation. You may find a class like this helpful: a way of getting your body moving in the company of others with the same uncertainties.

And read *Great Shape – the First Fitness Guide for Large Women* by Pat Lyons and Debby Burgard.[4] This will tell you everything you need to know about weight and fitness, sports physiology and psychology as applied to the large woman. It's excellent. Nobody should feel trapped in their body just because it is large. Move it!

Hunger and Satiety

'Never eat on an empty stomach' I used to tell my children, prompting any stray listeners to query whether I didn't mean 'on a *full* stomach'.

I did not. What I meant was don't let yourself get too hungry. *Extreme* hunger overrides the normal signals of appetite and in a seasoned dieter extreme hunger leads to body panic: 'This is famine, we've been here before and dreaded it happening again because it does us no good at all; quick, eat, stuff it in, all you can get before it disappears.' When people say they are famished, the linguistic proximity to the word 'famine' is not coincidental.

So, if you let yourself get very hungry on a weight-loss regime, the likelihood is that you will overeat. It's not greed; it's primevally driven need.

A few years ago I rescued a tiny ginger kitten from a farmer's barn. The farmer's wife had found him starving and she warned me that this kitten was constantly frantic for his food and I should be careful not to overfeed him because he did not know how to stop when he was full. I was astonished by the desperation of this little creature's famine response. When I fed him he gobbled his food so fast he frequently had bouts of loud hiccups which visibly shook his tiny body! Because we had other, grown-up cats, he learned to make a beeline for their food. Pushing them out of the way in his terrible anxiety, he would eat and eat until he was sick, or I came along and stopped him. Quite often when I picked him up his stomach was enormous, hard as a football and distended with excess food. And people are no different!

Part of the biological response to inadequate food supplies, whether from too rigorous dieting or local shortage, is that the mechanism that normally signals satiety fails. You don't know when you've had enough.

During World War II a group of young, healthy conscientious objectors volunteered for a study to monitor the effects of deprivation. For three months they ate normally, while their behaviour, eating patterns and personality were studied. Then their calorie intake was cut by half for a further three months.

The men could not stop talking and dreaming about food. Some planned to be chefs. Many found it impossible to keep to the diet and ate secretly. Their moods and behaviour changed; they became worried and depressed. They lost all sense of hunger and satiety. The physical and psychological effects of the deprivation lasted for many months after the experiment ended and some of the men felt they never really recovered from it.[5]

A similar, 'lifestyle' response to the same thing can be found in bulimics. You don't become bulimic unless you have had a period of starvation, whether from being anorexic or simply having lost weight through over-zealous dieting. When a bulimic binges, the amount of food eaten is phenomenal. The stomach has an enormous capacity to stretch and does so to accommodate obscene amounts of food – though the resultant discomfort would make anyone want to throw up. At the time of eating, though, the sufferer does not notice the distension; the food is forced down as fast as it will go. The following is a list of food eaten by a bulimic in one binge: two raw cauliflowers; two black puddings; one and a half pounds of raw liver; two pounds of kidneys; a piece of cheese; three pounds of raw carrots; two pounds of peas; a pound of mushrooms; ten peaches; four bananas; two apples; four pears; two pounds of plums; two pounds of grapes and some home-made bread.

The food was consumed over the course of one evening and the woman died from a ruptured oesophagus.[6] A bulimic in recovery phase will often eat 10–12,000 calories per day. Even in less excessive bouts of bulimic eating a woman may eat a couple of loaves of bread complete with butter and jam.

That should give some idea of the power of the body's starvation response. When you are trying to lose weight, don't get very hungry. There is no need. Eat small meals fairly often and make sure that whatever plan you follow is adequate in calories. Deprivation on a *good* diet will be to do with the type of food you eat, not the quantity.

Having said that, controlled voluntary hunger can be a pleasant feeling. If you allow yourself to feel the physical sensation of hunger, knowing that it is going to be satisfied soon by a meal that is both tasty and substantial enough, you can learn not only to bear physical hunger but to enjoy it. Most of us with a chequered dieting history have alternated between starving and being afraid to get at all hungry, so that we have lost the sensation of normal appetite. We experience 'mouth hunger', the desire to eat, but not the stomach rumbles of true hunger.

The 'appestat' in the brain – the mechanism that tells you when you've eaten enough – doesn't kick in until about twenty minutes after a meal. This is not some kind of evolutionary inefficiency, though it doesn't accord well with modern eating habits where meals are eaten quickly. In our forebears' time it took twenty minutes to chew through the hard grains and roots, the raw vegetables and the tough gristle from meat; they would have known when to stop while they were still eating.

The equivalent today is the leisurely meal with three courses so we would do better to emulate the French way of eating where they really 'make a meal of it'. A starter is a good idea for dieters because you will already have some feeling of satiety when you begin the main course and by the end of the meal you will know you have had sufficient.

Because your body will be anxious about getting enough food, it may not appear to take kindly to the smaller meals you are giving it. Try this, which works for me every time. If, at the end of a meal or a snack, you don't feel satisfied, tell yourself it's okay, you *can* have more, but not just yet. Say you'll go and do something else for twenty minutes or so and if you are still hungry then, you can come back and eat more. If you've planned this diet properly – that is, if you are eating sufficient calories to lose weight slowly but not so few that you lose it fast and are hungry – you will find you don't need the second helping.

There are bound to be occasional gnawing feelings: you need to remember that in order to lose weight you have to eat less than your body *needs*. Not less than you want, less than you actually need to maintain bodyweight. You have to undereat to create the negative energy balance necessary for losing weight. Alternatively, you have to exercise in a way that burns off sufficient calories to create that same negative energy balance. The ideal combination is moderate calorie reduction and increased energy output in a way that is sustainable for the rest of your life.

So you will sometimes feel hungry and that can make you feel anxious and restless, with your eye on the clock for the next meal. I cannot emphasise it too much so I'll say it again: *do not allow yourself to get very hungry*! If you do, it will get you down; you will feel you can't carry on, you'll blow it and get depressed. Hunger is the biggest cause of failed weight-loss attempts.

How to Eat on a Diet

The old three meals a day prescription is not ideal for the dieter: the gaps are too long and on a reduced calorie allowance you *will* feel hungry if you go for four or five hours without eating. Try four meals, or three meals and three snacks. My own pattern would bring a frown to the face of all those who believe in routine and regularity and no eating between meals, but it works for me and that is all that matters. I eat a piece of toast at 7 a.m., another at about 9.30 a.m., an apple at about 11 a.m. and lunch at 1 p.m. I have a snack at 3 p.m., another at 5 p.m and supper between 8 and 9 p.m. This is my own idiosyncratic timetable and it suits me. It is devised for the woman who has been on many diets before and who now has an ingrained anxiety response to hunger; who works at home alone all day and sometimes experiences the boredom that can lead to nibbling, so built-in snacks pre-empt that; in other words I've tailor-made it for me.

Not only does my diet prevent me from getting desperately hungry, it also provides opportunities for what Australian doctor Rick Kausman calls 'non-hungry eating'. Kausman is an acclaimed practitioner and author who has worked in the field of weight management and eating behaviour since 1987. His discourse on non-hungry eating cannot be bettered so I do not propose to deal with the subject in depth here but to direct you to his excellent book.[7]

Kausman points out that a significant amount of non-hungry eating leads to weight gain and that identifying the different types of this behaviour, and the reasons for it, is essential for weight loss. Once you recognise non-hungry eating for what it is, you can manage in a way that suits you and your diet – but that doesn't mean you have to stop it entirely. Because we live in an affluent society, and because eating is pleasurable, food has many more functions than that of simply satisfying hunger. Some people never indulge in non-hungry eating; most do and it can be a particular problem for women, for whom the issues around eating and food are often extremely complex.

I know that there are low points in my day when I want to eat for reasons not strictly to do with physical hunger. My diet has helped me to establish when those dips occur. I find I'm okay in the morning as long as I have the apple for elevenses. But afternoons often seem long and dreary so that's when I have my dried fruit. Between 5 p.m. and 6 p.m. is another difficult time, so that's why I have a snack then. After that I don't feel hungry in the physical or psychological sense for some time and can happily wait until 9 p.m. for supper.

The following exchange is an excellent example of non-hungry eating, one that is probably familiar to us all!

Child: I'm hungry.
Mother: Have a piece of bread.
Child: I don't want bread, I want some cake.
Mother: Then you're not hungry.

I was standing by the river the other day, waiting to see a display. Beside me was a woman with a little boy of about six. She was getting harassed by his constant requests for something to eat. 'He had a burger and chips on the way here,' she told me. 'Then I bought him some chocolate. And he's still hungry.' I told the mother that I had a banana and asked if she would like it for her little boy. She accepted gratefully. 'Do you like bananas?' I asked him. 'Yes,' he said. 'Would you like one?' I asked. 'No, thank you,' he said very definitely. He was not hungry, of course. I would guess he was very bored. Boredom and stress are huge triggers of non-hungry eating.

Jill Welbourne recommends this as a model for in-between-meals snacking: just eat for hunger, don't eat anything nice. I can see her point: if the food is tempting you might want a lot of it. Again it is something you have to work out for yourself: if your non-hungry snack is always a couple of dry rice cakes that take the edge of your appetite but give no real satisfaction, that may not do the trick. You might continue to prowl until you raid the biscuit tin because deep down you feel you have been deprived. Because dried fruit is one of my treats I use it for snacks (weighed on my calorie-counting scales because it would be too easy to dip into the packet and keep eating!).

It's important to allow yourself treats while dieting. Chocolate and alcohol are the two substances that most women feel they can't give up. No problem: just incorporate them into your allowance. But be careful. If you have a tendency to chocolate addiction, you may find that allowing yourself one small bar will be worse than avoiding it altogether. It can set up a longing and frustration that may drive you clean off your diet! It depends on the power of your own trigger foods and you need to take this into consideration when planning what to eat. If any particular food causes you to keep breaking out into a binge then don't have it in the house. It's hard enough losing weight without having to try to conquer addictions at the same time.

It is also essential that you don't get bored with what you are eating. It's all too easy to find something that works, that you can live with, that will *do*, and get locked into a dull routine of 'safe' foods. No good. Variety is vital, not only to avoid boredom but to make sure you get a wide range of nutrients. You need to plan tasty meals that are more than just a means to fuel your body or you will rebel. I'm all for rebellion in life, having been a natural non-conformist since birth, but I don't want to rebel on the diet. Because I chose to do it, I would be rebelling against myself, which would be somewhat counter-productive. What I do is try to make sure I have a delicious evening meal. That's when I eat the bulk of my calories – against the advice of all those who say you should dine like a pauper (having lunched like a prince, etc) – but knowing I've got that to come makes it easier to eat 'sensibly' during the day. I don't mind saving myself if there's something worth saving for.

The Food Diary

Keep a food diary. It's illuminating. Mine shows how I was able to eat far more calories – and lose weight – when I started the diet because I weighed so much more. It also shows that there have been periods of time when, although I have kept to the diet, I have not lost weight. Definite patterns emerge, which can be helpful when you are feeling stuck or hopeless. It also shows me at the moment that I really do have to be on a diet to maintain this weight, though it is less stringent than when I was losing.

The Counting Method

Some people absolutely hate the business of counting the food values of everything they eat. Others enjoy the sense of control it gives them, especially when they have had a chaotic dieting history. Calorie counting is really not difficult. Nearly every food from a pound of sausages to a pound of chocolate has its calorie value listed on the packaging. Even some pre-wrapped fruit and veg is calorie counted. For fresh foods there are plenty of cheap booklets to give you the values of those. You very quickly get to know them by heart and it is not the onerous task many anti-dieters make it out to be.

I really like my calorie-counting scales. Each food has a number: you put the food on the scales, key in the number and it tells you the weight and the number of calories. It may seem over-scrupulous but it's an eye opener. You pick up an apple and think 'one apple, 40 calories, that's what all the books say'. Apples, like everything else, are different sizes and weights. When I was eating an awful lot of apples (and estimating 40 calories for each one) I started to put on weight. When I acquired the scales I found that the apples I was eating were around 100 calories each and since I was eating six or seven a day, that made a difference.

But I will have no truck with the type of headmistressy dietitian who says you must weigh everything you eat and never eat more than 3 oz of chicken – or whatever – at one meal. That kind of restriction leads to rebellion and quite right too. Eat chicken breasts, salmon fillets, chops, lean mince – after a while you'll know their calorie value just by looking at them.

If you don't like the idea of calorie counting there are other methods: Weight Watchers Points and Slimming World Sins (see Chapter Ten: Don't Go it Alone for more details on these methods).

The Plate Method

This is Jill Welbourne's recommended method of restricting food intake for someone who has a considerable amount of weight to lose. You may prefer it to counting.

Buy a plate a size smaller than your usual dinner plate. You might find it useful to draw around your usual plate and take the piece of paper to the shop. Just one size down: about an inch smaller in diameter. Have four meals a day: breakfast within an hour of getting up, main meal at midday if possible, tea at 5.30 p.m. and supper at 9.30 p.m., never leaving more than about four hours between meals. If you can't manage that, have six half meals as long as the meals are evenly spaced and the same size. Each meal has to be balanced: equal amounts of protein and carbohydrate; smaller, but equal, servings of fruit and vegetables and a very small (half an ounce) amount of fat. Fill the plate in those proportions.

It doesn't matter what the food is as long as all the components are present. It can be six biscuits, one apple and a lump of cheese. The fat at breakfast can come from the nuts in muesli. Pay great attention to the quality of the food; use the best wholemeal bread, fresh fruit and vegetables, not frozen or tinned. Don't count calories. If after a week there is no change you may need to adjust to a smaller plate. Keep experimenting until the weight begins to come off slowly.

Like all weight-loss methods, this should be accompanied by exercise: nothing dramatic, just more use of stairs and a commitment to moving around as much as possible. Weight loss should be at the rate of $3/4$ lb per week. If it is any faster than that, you need to eat more.

The plate method would not suit everyone, but the point about weight loss is to find a method that feels okay for you. It could be a good method for those who are very strongly anti-diet but who really would like to lose weight. The fact that six biscuits and a piece of cheese can constitute a meal could make it an attractive proposition for those who don't want to eat what they consider to be 'diet food'. Obviously it works by portion control and therefore calorie reduction but if you don't have to count anything then it may feel less like being on a diet.

If you have a lot of weight to lose – if for example you weight 20 stone and you are aiming for 12 – Jill Welbourne suggests you stop for a break at 18 stone. Even that 10 per cent loss makes an enormous difference to health.

Put It in the Bin...

There are many, and I am one, who find wasting food almost a crime. These are usually the people who were brought up in poverty or who grew up during or just after World War II, when food was short and much was rationed. When you don't have enough to eat, when you have to make a meal out of the most unlikely scraps, you appreciate as we cannot now what a fundamental commodity food is. You never take it for granted. In the house of my childhood, as in many other homes up and down the land, the watchword was 'Waste not, want not'. (A semantic aside: 'want' was used in its original sense, meaning 'lack'. Its current sole meaning which relates only to gratification is a comment upon the times in which we live.) I can remember sitting in front of a half-finished bowl of soup feeling sick with every small spoonful I forced down, but I was not allowed to leave the table until it was finished.

Messages like these burn their way into the depths of our consciousness; powerful because in their most primitive sense they are about life and death. Food was never ever thrown away. There were always little bowls in the fridge or larder from which further meals could be made. The tiniest scraps were carefully hoarded. Soup can be made from the most disparate store cupboard contents. Anything really inedible went to feed the pigs or the hens. If you didn't clean your plate you were told you'd go hungry and that it was a long time till the next meal. Besides, cleaning your plate was a basic tenet of good manners so you were caught on all sides.

Because we are living in a time when food in an affluent society is actually *too* abundant, the impulse to put leftovers in the fridge to make another meal has lost its urgency. But those who grew up with these sorts of admonitions echoing through their brain will find it very hard to waste food, so a dilemma is created. Many overweight people solve this by feeling, consciously or otherwise, that they must finish all the food on their plates whether or not they have had enough. In doing so they may be taking in more than they need and it is by eating in this way over years that they have gained weight. It actually springs from an admirable intention and is far removed from the stereotypical social perception of the base motivations of the overeater.

Learning to leave food on my plate was one of the more testing parts of my weight-loss journey. Everything in me rebelled against it. I had always been horrified when my children – who like most of their generation have not been affected by the sort of food shortage mentality I grew up with – left food on their plates. Like so many mothers, I would finish it up for them, rather than see it go to waste. Even now I cannot help a mute cry of protest when, now grown up and with kitchens of their own, my children dump the remains of a meal unceremoniously into the bin instead of carefully decanting it into containers for the fridge.

But they have got it right because we are exposed to too much food, too many eating opportunities. We cannot any longer be guided by availability so we must be guided by appetite. 'Think of the starving millions in Africa' (another little homily we were subjected to) does not actually help the starving millions! Eating everything in sight on the grounds that we should be thankful that we have enough and they do not is counter-productive. The everyday products of our gastronomic excess do not result in direct deprivation to the starving. It is more complex than that.

There is a strong link between starving and overeating, particularly with eating everything in sight. I get very angry with those smug fat-bashers who say (always as though it were an original thought) 'Anyone can lose weight if they stop eating so much. After all, no one came out of Belsen fat.' No. They didn't. Or out of any other concentration camp or famine situation. But the people who did make it were those whose metabolisms were the most efficient, who were able to go into conserve mode, shut down all but the most essential metabolic processes and horde every available calorie and ounce of weight on their bodies. The deprivation suffered under those conditions is so appalling that few can survive it; of course they don't come out fat or even normal sized.

But when people survive extreme deprivation, they lose all sense of satiety. After starvation the most primitive, life-saving impulses are to feed the body with as much as is available. In a moderated form, these impulses are created when people follow a diet that is too low in calories, and most overweight people have done that at least once, probably many times. A permanent, underlying sense of apprehension pervades our attitudes to food; the body's constant, physical reminder that there have been times when it has been short-changed.

Bar Hewlett of *Obesity Lifeline* believes that the grab-it-all response is a result of infant-feeding schedules. If a baby is put on a strict three- or four-hour routine with no 'demand' feeding the chances are high that there will be periods of intense hunger and desperation because that hunger is not met. This, she believes, can set up a panic that drives us to keep eating. It's a plausible theory since babies' needs are elemental and I have no doubt that we carry within us deep memories of traumas experienced when we had no language to communicate our needs.

If you have a problem with leaving food, it is worth considering the possible origin of this. If it is constant and troublesome, if it sabotages your attempts to lose weight, it is likely that it has come from at least one episode of starvation, whether consciously remembered or not. Once you accept this to be the case, use a cognitive approach and tell yourself it is an inappropriate response. If you know that your stomach does not need that last slice of meat or two remaining potatoes, make a gargantuan effort, put down your knife and fork and *leave it*. It will call to you, that food, with all the power of the messages encoded in it. You will believe with every fibre of your being that you *must* eat it. The idea of not doing so can set up a dreadful sense of insecurity.

But this is all feeling; all pure emotion without logic. If you get caught in this trap (and believe me, I still do) just ask yourself some questions and make yourself answer them. Why do you want to eat that food when deep down you know you have had enough? Are you still hungry? Is it because it is something you particularly like? And finally (this one is the killer), what makes you think that food will be better off in your stomach than in the rubbish bin? If you can give a genuinely convincing answer to that last one, then you deserve the food and you probably need it.

You have to keep on the *qui vive* where this particular piece of discipline is concerned. When you're cooking your own meals at home it's not so bad because you can give yourself smallish quantities (and fend off looming feelings of anxiety by telling yourself you can always have second helpings after 20 minutes). But if you are out, there are other problems to cope with.

- You are eating at a friend's house. She has given you gigantic portions but it would be rude to leave the food she has slaved over. (*It wouldn't. You could either explain or leave a discreet little heap at the edge of your plate. You wouldn't be the only one in these diet-conscious times.*)
- You don't know when you'll get your next meal so you'd better stoke up. (*False logic. You can always plan eating times; it just requires a bit of attention to detail, which is boring. Carry a banana in your handbag for emergencies.*)

- You're in a restaurant and you have to eat everything in front of you because it is so delicious and it was so expensive. (*Delicious food is hard to resist, granted. But the expense is neither here nor there. You won't be doing yourself any favours by trying to get your money's worth: another piece of false logic.*)

I have a very overweight friend who has a great problem with the business of needing to consume something once it is paid for. If she's bought a theatre ticket she'll drive 20 miles on a winter's night with raging flu – because she's paid for it. If she buys a meal and there's a lot of it, she will eat it until her stomach is bulging and she's feeling none too good – because she's paid for it. She cannot understand the principle of food being better in the bin than in her stomach and her weight has steadily climbed over the years.

So, when faced with more on your plate than you need (or actually want, if you're really honest), steel yourself to chuck it.

What to Eat

A good balance of foods is more important on a weight-loss diet than it is normally because the restriction in calories means you will be eating less in the way of essential nutrients. Try to go for wholefoods of the best quality you can afford: organic if possible, but don't be purist over it.

Grains are an excellent food but don't stick to wheat and oats: health food shops have a huge range of the more unusual grains like millet and quinoa. Give them a try. Health food shops also have excellent preserves, jams made with whole fruit and no sugar at all. In fact, these stores have a number of foods not usually found on supermarket shelves which you might like to try.

Meat should be the leanest and best you can buy; fish should be fresh if possible. Fresh vegetables and fruit are essential: try to make sure you meet the World Health Organisation's Five-a-Day recommendation. Eat the full range of colours as each provides different vitamins: yellow peppers, beetroot, oranges, dark green leafy vegetables, green beans, tomatoes. Vary your diet as much as possible.

Pulses and pasta are good nutritious foods and are relatively low in calories. Eggs are excellent. As this is not a diet book I do not propose to go into menus in detail: these are meant to be just basic, common-sense guidelines.

If you like cooking there are some very inventive low-calorie cookbooks on the market. If you don't, there are ready meals. Don't rely too heavily on these, though. On the whole they are over-processed and too high in saturated fats and salt. I have to admit to eating a ready meal about twice a week and I see no harm in that. The rest of the time I cook chicken, fish, pasta, Quorn-based meals and vast vegetable stews.

Quorn products are a blessing for the dieter. Quorn is made from vegetable protein and is extremely low in fat and calories. You use it just as you would use meat: it comes in chunks and in mince. When it's wrapped in a sauce the most dedicated carnivore can't tell it from meat. Quorn also make wonderfully tasty things like Cheese and Broccoli En Croute with melting lattice pastry. Because Quorn is so low in calories – one large En Croute is only 317 – it is easily fitted into a dieter's allowance and is very satisfying.

What you really don't need to do is to buy purpose-made slimming meals, like Weight Watchers or Lean Cuisine. If you compare their calories and fat with other ready meals which are not specifically for dieters, there is often very little difference, if any. And the diet meals are frequently more expensive.

It is important to supplement your diet with a good one-a-day vitamin and mineral pill and an Omega 3 fish oil capsule. If you are vegetarian there are flaxseed oil capsules which provide the same essential fatty acids. If you have been assiduously avoiding fat, or conversely eating too much junk food, you will probably be short of efas and the capsule will help supply the deficit. If you are not a vegetarian, eat at least two helpings of oily fish a week.

When choosing what to eat on a diet, the main thing to remember is 'value for calories'. You can eat a great deal of the right food for 1500 calories per day. On the other hand, small amounts of high-calorie food use up your allowance and leave you feeling unsatisfied. The 3500 calories it takes to put on a pound of fat (not just weight – fat!) can be quickly and easily eaten in a high-fat, high-sugar meal. But it is not easy to cut back the 3500 calories to lose that pound of fat. Weight can be gained very fast indeed; losing it is another matter.

That's it really – the basic nuts and bolts of weight loss. Except – don't go it alone. Whether you are a group person or a loner, enlist somebody's help.

Chapter Ten
Don't Go It Alone:
The Importance of Support

The Lack of Individual Support

Losing weight alone, whether with a diet book, by counting calories or any other method you might choose, is very difficult indeed. You need someone in there with you, whether on a one-to-one basis or in a group. If you try to go it alone, the contrast between what you are doing and the eating behaviour of those who do not need or choose not to lose weight will make you feel envious, isolated or defiant. Weight loss in an affluent society that loves food is not a natural state to be in so you need someone to cheer you on and help you when the going gets tough.

Even the pundits, those obesity 'experts' who give us such a hard time, admit that one of the main causes of failure to lose weight, or maintain the loss, is lack of support.[1] In the sixties, when I went on the Big Diet for my wedding, my GP asked to see me every week and he weighed me himself. Because he was a good doctor, a kind man who really seemed to have my best interests at heart, this was a positive experience. I did feel supported by him and there is no doubt it helped me to maintain my focus. If I flagged, got despondent, or broke my diet, the weekly check-in got me back on course. But the days when a doctor would or could take such an interest in a patient's weight problem are long gone.

Considering that the medical profession and bossy government departments like the National Audit Office are so down on the overweight, they provide very little in the way of useful, productive support. The first port of call for someone who wants to lose weight and would like a helping hand is usually the GP. There is a token move now towards providing back-up for the dieter, but it is counter-productive because it is temporary. Many surgeries now adopt a three-pronged approach to the patient who asks for help with weight loss. They will be referred to the practice dietitian if there is one. They may be able to talk to the practice counsellor if it is considered that there is a psychological component to their weight problem. And – the latest thing – they may be prescribed a limited number of sessions at the local gym or fitness centre. Carried along on a cushion of nice, positive motivation, they start losing weight. Then the sessions with the helpful professionals dry up; they're on their own.

Think of it. You're on a weight-loss regime of some kind and you run into difficulties. Or perhaps you have questions. Your weight plateaus even though you're still following your diet. Or you feel hungry all the time. Or any one of a hundred different things. Whom do you ask? You've finished seeing all those people the doctor set you up with: you're not entitled to any more sessions. You can't keep going to the GP. Even if you did, it's doubtful s/he would be able to help.

I think this is outrageous. If people were permitted to be fat this lack of help and support would not be so bad. If 'they', the ever present, punishing authorities, said: 'Overweight? No problem. Just eat healthily, exercise moderately and enjoy life. No, of course you won't be discriminated against. Of course medical treatment will not be conditional on your losing weight. We're all equal in this society,' – as I said, *if* this were the case the lack of support for those who wanted to lose weight would not be such a scandal. But honest medical professionals admit that permanent weight loss is one of the most difficult things to achieve even with support. When you are losing weight alone, or with only temporary support, it is almost impossible. Susan Jebb of the Association for the Study of Obesity (ASO) states that trials show that the often-quoted 95 per cent regain figure is accurate and that difficulties arise when support is withdrawn. People lose motivation and weight regain is the biggest problem in weight control. She believes that there should be full resources for people who want to lose weight and that support is crucial.[2] But it is not there.

When I asked Dr Julian Barth (the good guy who treats obesity at Leeds General Infirmary) why these clinics had such a poor success rate, he explained that there are only eight obesity clinics in the entire country and they have long waiting lists. Because resources are so scarce they can only help the most intractable cases. Usually, these are people whose life events have been so unbearable, who have been in so much pain and despair, that their only recourse is to eat, just as others might drink or turn to drugs, sex, gambling or simply opting out. In the case of many of the patients, he said, 'the impulses to eat cannot be overridden.'[3]

This is a welcome admission from two members of the medical fraternity working in the field of obesity research and treatment. They are not blaming the fat person – a rare and precious event! But they are underlining the huge problem of the paucity of support. If some of the medical profession, then, can admit that both obesity and difficulty with permanent weight loss are not the fault of the individual, should the whole lot of them not shut up until they can provide something worthwhile in the way of understanding, treatment, compassion and support? If only.

What does tend to happen is that, pressured by the government, various task forces, the WHO, the NAO and a lot of other organisations with initials, our desperate doctors resort to unsafe and largely ineffectual drugs and surgery. Surely it would be cheaper to set up a nationwide support system for those who want to lose weight? Or is that too simple?

Group Support

The efficacy of group support has been most dramatically proven by the success of Alcoholics Anonymous. Alcoholism is one of the most intractable illnesses there is and doctors and therapists have little idea of how to treat it. An AA meeting, though, is an extraordinary dynamic powerhouse. The group energy works in a vital and rather mysterious way that makes it apparent that it is more than the sum of its parts. People can and do recover from alcoholism for life, even though an alcoholic will never say he or she is cured. Anyone who has recovered through AA will attest to the fact that they could not have done so without the group. They will also affirm that if they leave AA the chances that they will start to drink again are very high. Whether it's drink, drugs or weight loss that's the issue, recidivism is far less likely when there is group support.

There is a number of slimming organisations that hold group meetings; I propose to talk about the three best known. The principles are the same: support, a degree of competition, practical advice and the sharing of information and experience. All require some form of counting: calories, fat grams, sins or points. There's no magic here: like all diets, each group's 'plan' is about limiting calorie intake. I was amused when talking to representatives from every organisation to find that each one disparages the other's method as being 'too complicated' or requiring 'so much effort'. In the end they are all the same; some basic arithmetic is needed to calculate food values.

None of the organisations holds records of long-term success though there is a good deal of informal evidence to show that staying as a member, even when the target weight has been achieved, gives the best chance of maintaining weight loss.

Slimming World

Many people, including those running other weight-loss organisations, mistakenly think the Slimming World method is about food combining and so find it off-putting. This is because the eating plan consists of Red (officially called Original) and Green days. Choices on Red days are mainly meat and fish; on Green days it's pasta, pulses, grains and unlimited root vegetables. However, this does not preclude meat and fish on Green days, nor grains on Red. It's a matter of preponderance. Obviously if you stuffed yourself with pasta and had half a chicken on the side, weight loss would be somewhat elusive.

The Slimming World plan is called Food Optimising: a rather unwieldy term beloved by the hierarchy though not often used by class members. There are three categories in the eating plan, from which you draw each day: free foods, healthy extras and sins.

Healthy extras are compulsory. They are measured servings of a variety of foods containing fibre and/or vitamins and minerals. You choose any two of these each day: a serving of cereal or bread, dried fruit, milk, cheese, fish, meat, nuts – a very long list. The reason for this is to ensure you have a healthy, nutritious, balanced diet with no shortages of essential foods.

Free foods are what makes the Slimming World method so successful, though in many ways the free-food concept defies logic. It means that you can eat unlimited quantities of a huge range of foods – not just green vegetables and stock cubes, either. The list includes all meat and fish (on Original days) and all grains, pulses and pasta (on Green days). There is also a large number of branded foods, some of which would appear to have no place on a diet, like curries, macaroni cheese and things in creamy sauces. The psychology of the free-food principle is excellent. It means you need never be hungry and, because many of the foods are satisfying, it minimises the feelings of deprivation. The only snag is that as your basal metabolic rate drops along with your weight loss you may not be able to get away with eating free foods freely. In the end calories do count, unfortunately.

People often query the free-food allowance; I was one of them. There are some nice high-calorie comfort foods on the list. And surely, people say, you can't eat a whole chicken and lose weight? What if you binge on macaroni cheese? The answer is that because the foods are allowed without restriction, people tend to self-limit. If you are used to severely limited diets you may break out and eat a large quantity of free foods at first. I can remember eating two tins of baked beans or tinned pasta meals in one go when I first joined Slimming World, but I didn't need to do so very often, and when I did, it meant that I wasn't hungry for a long time afterwards. Most diets fail because there comes a point in the day when you have used up your calorie or points allowance; the only thing left to eat doesn't satisfy you and you break out with a binge through sheer hunger.

The free-food system satisfies those dieters who don't want to think they are restricting their calorie intake, and those practitioners, like Jill Welbourne, who believe that counting calories is the way to disaster.

Sins are high-calorie foods to which Slimming World allots a numerical value. Thus a chicken Kiev has seven-and-a-half sins, a Cadbury's creme egg has eight-and-a-half. You have a sin allowance of 10 a day or 70 a week. Another good piece of psychology is Flexible Sins. This means that if you have a day out, a special occasion, or you just want to eat as much as you want and blow the diet, you do so but keep count of the sin values. You may notch up 100 sins in a day, but the thinking is that as long as you *count* them you are keeping control rather than bingeing in a meaningless way. The following day you go back to your normal 10 sin count – you don't have to 'pay' for the Flexible Sin day. Counting sins, even if they mount up, means that a day off the diet doesn't mean you feel you've wrecked it. Because you're still counting, you don't feel you've lost control; you feel in charge of your eating and not that food is in charge of you.

Slimming World classes tend to be very informal and friendly. There is the weigh-in followed by Image Therapy, another fancy name which means sharing experiences and having a chat with the class consultant. Weight losses and gains are read out (though not actual weights). Members are praised and/or encouraged. No one is made to feel a failure. Hints, tips, failings, successes and recipes are exchanged. Slimming World recipes are excellent: they have a low-calorie cheesecake and a tiramisu, neither of which would be out of place at a smart dinner party. Sin-free chips (sprayed with a fine mist of oil and cooked in the oven) are a great favourite: on Green Days potatoes are a free food which means you can eat a huge plate of chips with sin-counted fish fingers and tomato ketchup.

As at Weight Watchers, praise is given to those with large weight losses. Class consultants do not have to have reached their target weight, though they will continue to attend another class as a member. Some are still struggling and in many ways this makes them more human and approachable.

One excellent thing about Slimming World is that you set your target weight in steps. For example, if you go along there weighing 15 stone with a chequered dieting history, fear in your heart and doubt in your mind, then the thought of losing five stone is hugely daunting. So you can set a half stone goal or any amount you like.

Weight Watchers

I've been to Weight Watchers twice: once when I was in my late teens and again in my early thirties. My experience of it was that it was rather punitive. In those days, you were shamed and rebuked in front of the whole class if you put on weight. I suppose the idea was that you would rush home full of fresh resolve and the prospect of further humiliation would help you stick to the diet. My memory is that Weight Watchers was full of Don'ts and things that were strictly forbidden.

It is not like that now, though compared to Slimming World it is still authoritarian. Weight Watchers would not do for renegades like me since they don't allow you to set your own goal weight. Weight Watchers' goal weights come within the recommended BMI – that damned set of initials that dogs anyone with even a passing interest in their weight (and what woman has less than a passing interest in it, whatever form that interest may take?). So, for instance, the very most that I would be allowed to be, to make my body mass acceptable, is 10 stone 1 lb. But time, circumstances and my own particular preference combine to make that an unattainable weight for me. The very lowest I should like to be is 11 stone. I actually think that is an unrealistic goal, so I'd be happy to be 12. The reality, though, is that in middle age and with a long dieting history, I am unlikely now to go much below 13.

The end result of losing weight in a class – the bonus, the prize – is that when you've achieved your target you can maintain it with the support of the group without paying the weekly fee. This is true of Weight Watchers, too. You can attend as a Gold member as long as you don't weigh more than 5 lbs above your goal, but you have to get down to the goal first. As I don't want to reach 10 st 1 lb I would have to continue to pay the weekly fee, so Weight Watchers is not for those of us who will not accept having our weights dictated.

The Weight Watchers' Points system, which allocates a value to each food, is based on a daily calorie allowance of about 1250 calories. Heavier members may start the diet on a higher calorie/points allowance because of the greater calorific requirement of the large body. I think it unlikely that many people would be able to maintain a daily intake of only 1250 calories without being hungry.

Like Slimming World, Weight Watchers members are given much praise if they lose a great deal of weight in a week – anything from 3 lbs upwards. At the class I observed, the member who said she was going for a 4 lb loss by the following week was much encouraged by the leader. This is in spite of the fact that a weight loss of more than 2 lbs a week is neither healthy nor usually sustainable. Weight Watchers point out that these losses do not tend to occur regularly but even out, so the average weight loss is nearer to what is reasonable.

The point of this kind of encouragement to lose fast is simple. Slimming clubs make a great deal of money and are in competition with each other. Women, however much they read or are told that slow weight loss is sensible and healthy, do not usually want slow weight loss. They want something that will enable them to lose 4 lbs a week. As a Weight Watchers spokesperson put it to me: not many people would be motivated if they were told they were only going to lose half a pound a week.[4] Yet half a pound a week is probably the best and healthiest weight loss of all and the one which gives you the greatest chance of keeping the weight off. As discussed earlier, there are two good reasons for this: if you are only losing half a pound a week, you will still be eating a reasonable number of calories so you won't be hungry and you are less likely to 'break the diet' or binge. In addition, the slow weight loss is less likely to cause your body to leap into famine alert and to put your metabolism into 'conserve mode'.

But this is a business, a business with huge profits. If losses of 3 lbs or more per week are going to bring the punters on board – and they will, the spokesperson was right – then such losses will not be discouraged.

Weight Watchers 'leaders' have to reach goal weight before they can be considered for training and they have to maintain goal weight while they are working for the organisation. If the idea of being a Weight Watchers leader appeals – and there's no doubt it does to some women – then it's probably a good motivational force for maintaining weight loss. The leader of the class I observed had maintained her four-stone loss for three years.

The class consisted of the weigh-in, with encouragement for those who had lost and words of wisdom for those who had not. It was interesting to see that the one male member of the class was far more laid-back than any of the women and, unlike them, he kept his jumper on. They stripped off as far as they dared, and I admit to having done the same myself. Ridiculous, ludicrous, but everyone wants to see a loss. Common sense should tell us that as long as we wear roughly the same clothes every week it doesn't matter how heavy they are. But people even take their watches off – anything that they think could possibly influence the scales.

Here's a tip: just before you get weighed, exhale forcefully and hold your breath. That way you will lose the weight of the air that would otherwise have been in your lungs. (And if you believe that, Father Christmas is alive and well and living in Lapland. Though undoubtedly some women would give it a try.)

After the weigh-in the leader gave a lecture. She asked if anyone was disappointed with their weight. Sometimes, she said, you could be doing everything right and not have a good weight loss but don't worry, it will show the next week. If you want a treat you should have it, not deny yourself or you'll eat more. Suggestions were made about fish and chips, seemingly a particular favourite. Have the fish without batter, said one woman, or have a children's portion, suggested another. 'I have fish and chips every single week,' said one, silencing the class for a moment. 'You can have anything you want as long as you count points,' advised the leader. I stared at a poster with a slogan on it: 'Knowing your trigger will stop you getting bigger'. Not bad advice.

The leader put up the word 'activate' and members were invited to use it as an acronym and suggest the most appropriate words for each letter. C of course was cheating. E was exercise, envy, enthusiasm and euphoria. I wanted to suggest that eating was a fairly important word to bear in mind but felt I'd better not as I was not a class member.

There were confessions. Cheating was probably the word, along with 'good', most used amongst the slimmers. 'Has anyone got a goal?' asked the leader. Holidays seemed to be the thing: to lose so much weight before they came around. There was a kind of temporary feel to that, as though once the holiday had been and gone the weight didn't matter so much.

Finally, the class's aggregate weight loss for that week was announced: 55 lbs. 'That's more than a pound a week,' said the leader triumphantly. 'Next week I want it to be sixty.'

There's nothing intrinsically wrong with the Weight Watchers diet except that it is on the lean and hungry side and therefore less likely to result in a permanent loss. There were a number of Weight Watchers 'casualties' in my Slimming World class.

Rosemary Conley Diet and Fitness Classes

These are part of the multi-million pound Rosemary Conley organisation. No points or sins here, but calories and fat grams are counted. The main emphasis is on low-fat eating and exercise.

I went to meet Rosemary Conley, quite sure I wouldn't take to her. I am 13 stone, unfashionable and often dishevelled, with unstyled hair. Rosemary is very thin (seven and a half stone), smartly dressed, made-up, with a rigid blonde coiffure. Rosemary was desperately unhappy at her highest weight of 10 st 3 lbs. I would feel like a sprite at that weight. We are the same height. What could we possibly have in common?

I liked her. Though she is obviously a sharp businesswoman, though she has made immense amounts of money through a clever idea, I found her warm and friendly. And – shoot me down in flames, all you to whom any part of the diet industry is as acceptable as the Ku Klux Klan – I believe she cares about her clients. I cannot find fault with the ethics of what she is doing. She is providing a service that people want and because so many people want it she makes a lot of money. Can she be blamed for that? I don't think so. I think slimming clubs provide a reputable and reasonably priced service for the thousands of women who want to lose weight.

In her own words: 'The diet industry is crying out for somebody with some integrity who will actually say that people do need help, and we're prepared to help them honestly. I do care. I reply to people's letters, I'll send them a book, give advice. People need help and I remember what that was like.'

Rosemary Conley is not a serial dieter. She joined a slimming club when she weighed 9 stone 3 lbs (why? I hear you cry; it was my cry too but she didn't like being 9 stone 3 lbs.) She lost a stone, stopped attending and did a cordon bleu cookery course during her first marriage. Her weight shot up to 10 stone 3 lbs, a gain of two stone. This was her lowest – or highest – point. 'I absolutely hated myself,' she said. 'I get a lot of flak for that because people think that weight is nothing. But it was 25 per cent more than I wanted to be. I knew I was happy at 8 stone.' She is even happier at $7^1/_2$ stone, a weight she says she has achieved because her appetite has changed.

She devised her own diet, got down to $8^1/_2$ stone and started her own classes with the – surely not unintentional – acronym SAGG: Slimming and Good Grooming. After eight years, she sold out to IPC. She had written three books and then came the point at which the Hip and Thigh Diet came into being and made her fortune. She had had gallstones, was told to go on a low-fat diet to avoid surgery and lost 6 lbs from her hips and thighs. 'When I hit the big time I was ready for it,' she said.

Apart from her phobia about dietary fat, her nutritional principles are sound, though some of her earlier recipes were very heavy on sugar. She's very hot on the idea that you should not feel deprived:

I'm against buying low-sugar baked beans. Ordinary baked beans are fine. That's not where the badness is: the badness is going and having a burger and chips. And you mustn't be hungry or you're not going to stick to it. When someone is trying to lose weight you need to give them more food not less. These people are overweight because they've overeaten. And you have to accept there are people out there who just love food too much. They can't help it; they wish they didn't.

Rosemary Conley used to advocate a daily calorie allowance of 1400 but now her class instructors calculate each person's requirement based on their resting metabolic rate. This makes much more sense as there is no one-size-fits-all diet. For instance, a 33-year-old woman weighing 15 stone needs 1639 calories at rest. As soon as she gets up she requires more, so if she went on a diet of 1600 calories per day she would lose weight.

She knows about the dangers of crash dieting and recommends a loss of 1–2 lbs per week. To lose more than that is false economy, she says, and will cause more of a problem in the long run.

Conley has lots of advice about how to manage social eating, like not having seconds, and watching slim people to see how they eat. 'People sometimes feel food is the enemy,' she says. Many women who have struggled with cycles of dieting and regain feel food has far more power than they do themselves. She also makes some startling observations:

At lunchtime, in an environment where people are trying to lose weight, their appetites are so much greater than that of a normal person. When we do roadshows we may have 300 people. Any catering organisation knows how to cater for 300, except when those people belong to a slimming club and they eat much more so you have to tell the caterers that we need one-and-a-half portions per person, or you run out of food. That's because people who have to watch their weight have bigger appetites in the first place.

I think what she means is that people are fat because they overeat. In a literal sense that's true though, as Julian Barth pointed out, 'overeat' is best avoided because of its heavy moral and judgemental overtones. But unless someone has one of the rare metabolic or hormonal disorders (what they always used to refer to as 'glandular'), weight is gained because the body is in positive energy balance: too many calories in and too few going out. Do the people she refers to, the ones that have to be over-catered for, eat too much because their appetites are naturally too large, or because they are responding with the diet-induced starvation response? Perhaps we shall never know. Rosemary Conley herself admits to having been a binge eater, though it's hard to take that seriously: 'I would have three bowls of cornflakes, I'd have three rounds of toast. I'd eat cooking chocolate, all sorts of stuff, so I was a binge eater, definitely, so I know what people go through.'

Her classes differ from the other two organisations in that they incorporate a 45-minute workout with a trained fitness instructor. Conley is very keen on the group therapy aspect, on the importance of praise – a round of applause when weight is lost.

Support in weight loss is important because dieting is so difficult; there are hurdles and pitfalls and stumbling blocks along the way. 'If you have a support system in place it helps stop despair,' says Rosemary Reed of Slimming World. 'Other people can suggest things you might not have thought of and there is always someone at the end of the phone. There *are* times when you feel desperate, and that's when people trying to do it on their own often give up.'

Chapter Eleven
Troubleshooting:
When the Going Gets Tough

No pain, no gain – or in this case, loss. There will be times when you *hate* the fact that you are on a diet. You will experience a weakening of spirit, a lassitude; sometimes you may feel that it just isn't worth it. You will long to go back to normal eating. You will be fed up with counting, planning, excluding, balancing and being constantly watchful.

And these feelings can strike when the diet is going *well*. When it seems to be going badly you will probably feel like throwing in the towel. I know; I've trodden this particular path for nearly three years. Dieting troubles may come 'not as single spies but in battalions'. When they do, you need your troubleshooting armoury at the ready. There *is* a way through all these difficulties.

Plateauing

A cardinal rule of weight loss: expect the plateaus. A weight-loss graph should not look like the descent from a mountain: it should resemble a flight of stairs. Unfortunately it's the one thing a dieter doesn't want to see: you stick to the diet and there's no change – or worse, you've gained a pound or two. It can be disheartening to say the least.

It's partly because most people on diets weigh themselves weekly. Weight can fluctuate by several pounds during the course of a week, or even a day, but weigh yourself at the same time seven days later and you may have lost, or still be the same. True weight loss is better gauged over the course of a month, not a week. So if you're the same weight three weeks running, you may lose 3 lbs during the fourth. There are often time lags. Just because we tend to talk about weight loss in weekly units does not mean that our bodies have to comply. Weight loss has its own mysterious biochemistry and in women it is tied up with the menstrual cycle, too. It's unreasonable to expect a steady, consistent loss. Plateaus are normal. They are the body's way of adjusting to the fact that it is being consumed – like us it needs time to stop and think about changes that are being demanded of it.

When you first start a diet you'll experience a pretty big loss in the form of stored fluid. I lost 10 lbs in my first week. It's nice to feel things are shifting so quickly but it doesn't go on like that; the next week you may lose nothing. Don't get high on that initial loss and, whatever you do, don't aim for further big losses. I know about all the hype and glory in slimming clubs when someone records a 5 lb loss: the sharp intakes of envious breath, the applause, the praise, the smirk (or the amazement) on the face of the dieter. It's difficult not to feel smug, but if you've lost that much you've lost either essential lean tissue or fluid or a combination of both. It's counter-productive.

My first small plateau appeared in my fifth week. After I had lost a stone and a half, more small plateaus occurred fairly frequently. By the time I'd lost two stone, I was plateauing for longer periods. What emerges, looking at my chart, is a definite pattern of plateaus followed by several weeks of slow, steady loss. But the more weight I lost, the longer the plateaus lasted (remember your body will fight to resist the depletion of its tissue and you can't beat biology, no matter how hard you try). After I had lost four stone it became very hard indeed. It took three and a half months to lose the next half stone. The biggest plateau of all came between four and five stone: I reached 15 stone on 1 February and 14 stone on 17 October. The next stone, to my current weight of 13 stone, took seven months. It's because of those ever-lengthening periods of plateau that I know my body needs a break, that it doesn't want to lose any more of itself.

At the time, it feels awful and I have to admit you get very despondent. You're keeping to a diet, going through all the denial and deprivation, and week after week your weight sticks. There was one patch where I didn't shift a single pound for four whole months. You could be forgiven in these circumstances for thinking dieting really doesn't work and giving the whole thing up.

And of course this is one of the causes of diet failure: the inability or reluctance to accept that plateaus – long plateaus – are part of a normal weight-loss pattern. You feel despairing, defiant and bloody fed up. It's not working, you think, so bang goes the diet. Plateaus – seemingly intractable plateaus – are one of the key factors which separate the 95 per cent from the 5 per cent. You have to hang in there.

The course of weight loss never will run smooth: after all, it's against Nature. But there are things which will help you over plateaus.

How to Get Off a Plateau
Variety in the Diet

I have no scientific evidence or explanation for this strategy but I do know that changing what you eat can shift you off a plateau. It is very easy to get stuck on the same trusted foods, the ones that fill you up but have in the past kept the weight loss going, or at least don't cause you to put it back on again. If you look at what you are eating and change as much as you can you'll probably start to lose again but only if your body is ready to do so.

Protein to the rescue

Eat more and make it protein. Protein has a 'specific dynamic action' which means that you use more energy (calories) to digest it. The metabolism is a fire and it requires fuel; if it gets too low it will not burn efficiently. Protein is like throwing on a couple of good dry logs. But this is not to advocate one of the wacky, high-protein diets; they are a different matter altogether and are not recommended at all. But four days or so of increased protein at every meal will get your metabolism carrying out heat-producing reactions and will kick-start it into burning fat. This should be first-class protein: milk, eggs, lean meat and fish. Don't use cheese: it is a high-fat food and therefore extremely calorie dense.

Although some nutritionists list nuts and soya as first-class protein, Jill Welbourne asserts that for weight loss it really does need to be first-class animal protein. Sorry, vegans.

Exercise

Exercise speeds metabolism because exercise requires energy. Increase it when you plateau but not a huge amount or you won't be able to keep it up. The trick is to do just enough to make a difference but not so much that you start losing weight faster than you were. Even though plateaus are immensely frustrating, the aim should still be to continue losing weight slowly, not to speed it up to make up for the weeks you haven't lost anything.

Boredom, Apathy and Other Troublesome Feelings

There is something relentless about being on a diet, though it need not be boring, just restrictive. It has to be said that there are masses of good diet cookbooks with ingenious recipes which really are good enough (almost) to make you feel you're not dieting, though the portions may seem a bit meagre. Variety is essential and if you like cooking or, better still, have someone to cook for you, it's a breeze. (Though when Oprah Winfrey used to talk about her personal chef and the cordon bleu diet delights she came up with, I used to think enviously that anyone could lose weight and keep it off if they were being served that kind of food. But Oprah didn't.)

So keep changing what you eat. Although I don't like cooking, one of the bonuses of this diet has been that I have discovered new things. I also buy food that I would have considered too expensive before, like exotic fruits. I now have a passion for sharon fruit that outstrips my former passion for chocolate.

But there's another kind of boredom: the *tedium vitae* sort where everything just looks bleak. It's not exactly depression but it's a fairly close relative. You're not enjoying work, the weather is getting you down, there's nothing exciting on the horizon, you feel sluggish and unmotivated. There's no spark and all is definitely not right with the world. What would make it all better, you think, would be to have something nice to eat and plenty of it. It's one of those scenarios where non-dieting women buy chocolate.

So buy chocolate. Or cake. Just have a day when you forget the diet. Eat what it is you've been wanting to eat. But take control of it. Decide what you are going to have and how much – if it's half a pound of chocolate or three doughnuts, fine. Have enough to satisfy all the deprived feelings. If you want a large bar of chocolate don't buy a small one. Sit down, relax and enjoy it. Savour it. Don't binge in that altered-state-of-consciousness-wrapped-in-guilt way that is characteristic of out-of-control eating. Be in charge of your binge. Be mindful and aware in a zen kind of way. But only do it for one day.

I'm all for the occasional controlled binge. It's an emotive word, associated as it is with pathology and greedy fat people, but it's what 'normal'-weight people often do. It's just that they incorporate it into their lives without guilt or the opprobrium of society. If you don't do it when you desperately feel you need to, the urge will hang around and you probably *will* give in, though by then it won't be controlled. Whatever you eat on your binge – let's call it a feast – one day is not going to scupper your weight loss. Even a 'binge' of several days, like Christmas or a holiday, results in a good deal of fluid gained as weight; this is usually lost as quickly as it was gained as long as you go back to the diet.

Eating, which does no one any harm except perhaps the eater when it all goes wrong, carries connotations so loaded with danger and disapproval that someone from a less affluent culture could be forgiven for thinking we have lost all sense of judgement. Drinking alcohol, on the other hand – something which kills thousands of people every year and wrecks lives and families – is, on the whole, seen as pretty cool and certainly desirable. People will boast about what they drank last night; they will deliberately go and get drunk, announcing their intention beforehand and reporting on it afterwards. An excess of alcohol, with its real dangers and its countless working days lost through hangovers, is an acceptable part of social life. Excess eating never is, unless you are thin, in which case it is admired because you can eat and not get fat.

Emotional Eating

This is a whole book in itself and overlaps with the area of eating disorders. However, eating for emotional reasons does not necessarily mean disordered eating; most women do it at some time. But in the context of a diet, emotional eating can be the saboteur of successful weight loss.

Because it is such a huge subject I need to simplify it for the purposes of this book. As a generalisation, most large women have had a problem at some time with emotional eating. This includes: picking at food because you are bored or because your life is not the way you would like it to be; eating under stress and pressure; and comfort eating. For some, the problem cannot be solved just by undertaking a weight-loss programme because the underlying emotional issues cannot be dealt with simply by reducing calorie intake.

There are practical ways to deal with emotional eating. When you feel the need to eat, try to tune in to what that need feels like. A history of emotional eating can mean that you feel 'hungry' even though your body is satisified: it is another type of hunger you are feeling. Ask yourself if you really need food as fuel. If you have allowed yourself to feel some controlled physical hunger on your diet, hunger which you satisfy before you become ravenous, you should fairly easily be able to identify the nature of your need to eat.

If it is not physical hunger, it may still be a strong urge: mouth hunger rather than stomach hunger. You want the feel, the taste, the texture and the satisfying physical action of eating. Try to listen to what your body is telling you. If you can put to one side the voice in your head that says 'I want something to eat and I want it now,' you will get other messages, ones that can locate the nature of the need. Sometimes having a drink helps; sugarless tea, coffee, herb tea or a diet drink. I have never found that diet drinks have stimulated my appetite or my desire for sugar, though I am not happy about the chemicals they contain.

It helps to identify times in the day when you are prone to snacking. I have found that non-physical hunger does disappear if I go and immerse myself in something at those times, even if it is something I'm not particularly keen to do. Just the action of doing it helps. If I'm genuinely not hungry, telling my body that it doesn't need food now but can have some soon does the trick. If you are prone to emotional eating, the three meals and three snacks eating timetable will probably suit you best because there are never long foodless gaps.

It may sound over-simplistic, but identifying the areas in your life which are making you unhappy or over-stressed and taking appropriate action can put an end to out of control emotional eating. If it is an intractable problem – if you feel that the need to eat is so desperate that even a generous diet will not work for you – then you may want to seek professional help. But above all, don't blame yourself.

Night-eating Syndrome

Some people can't sleep because they keep thinking about food. Others get up in the night, maybe as many as five or six times, go downstairs and raid the fridge or the larder. They are not really awake, they are in a semi-sleepwalking condition. They often don't remember anything about it and come down in the morning to find that they've raided the custard powder, or something equally bizarre. People in this state, says Jill Welbourne, are drawn to calorie-dense or high-fat food: the sort of food they won't let themselves eat during the day.

> It comes from going to bed hungry. People suffering from this don't eat enough. They think they do but they are trying to live on under 1000 calories a day, which isn't enough to fuel anyone for a busy life. This behaviour takes place when the superego – the rulemaking part of your brain – is out of action, because it's fuzzy with sleep, so it can't stop you having the food you actually need but don't permit yourself to have.

> Although not particularly common, night-eating syndrome is found more in the overweight than in those of average weight. There is a theory that sufferers of night-eating syndrome have a deficiency in leptin, the hormone that switches off appetite, but Jill Welbourne thinks it is a specific kind of deficiency: 'The pattern of leptin secretion is shaped by training. For instance, people who miss breakfast can't afford to have high levels of leptin at night because otherwise they wouldn't get enough to eat.'
> Night-eating syndrome is a by-product of low-calorie dieting. It is not a mysterious eating disorder. There is a simple cure. It's another bit of evidence that low-calorie dieting never works.

Hungry Days

Some days you feel more hungry – physically hungry – than others and you will be more conscious of it than non-dieters. If you feel hungry, eat. Everyone experiences fluctuations in the degree of hunger they feel. If you are worried about blowing the diet, then let me assure you that you are far more likely to do so if you don't respond to your hunger. If you try to put up with it you'll end up eating out of desperation and probably eat more than if you'd listened to your body in the first place.

Only the body knows why it is hungrier some days than others. It happened to me this week: I'd eaten breakfast, lunch and tea in the normal way but had felt hungry throughout the day. So I had something extra after lunch, and a larger than usual snack in the afternoon. Then I had something at teatime. By seven o'clock I was famished and feeling all the symptoms of low blood sugar: dizziness, disorientation, etc. I needed more at supper than I usually have, so I had more. Over all I must have eaten at least 500 calories more that day than I usually do. The next day my hunger was back to normal. If I had not satisfied my appetite, I would have been hungrier still the next day – and persistent hunger inevitably leads to a binge.

It's important not to panic when you have hungry days, not to feel that perhaps your appetite is increasing and that if you give in to it you'll put on weight. If you *don't* give in to it you'll put on weight; that's a certainty. When I talk about dieting entailing denial and deprivation, I don't mean going hungry.

The Unpleasant Effects of a Lowered Metabolic Rate

As I write this in July the sun is shining and people are wandering around mopping their sweaty brows and saying 'I like it hot but not this hot.' Now I'm not saying that I'm cold, though I am wearing a cardigan while everyone else is stripped to the minimum; I feel thermostatically comfortable. But since losing six and a half stone, feeling cold has been real misery. When I am warm enough in the house, my husband sits wearing only his boxer shorts. I thought he was making a fuss until I saw the sweat running down his face. Cries of 'You *can't* still be cold' are answered by '*You* can't be hot.' Fortunately, we can both see the funny side.

Overweight people aren't supposed to feel the cold because of all the subcutaneous fat: the stuff that would stop us dying from hypothermia while our thinner friends perished. At 13 stone I must have a good layer of it still but I am freezing. It's because I now have a reduced metabolic rate and my efficient body is not going to spend its limited resources keeping me warmer than is essential to life. (I feel it's essential to *my* life but my body doesn't see it like that. 'You ain't at risk of hypothermia,' it tells me. 'Stop whingeing.')

My body temperature and blood pressure are very low and my heartbeat is slow. All these symptoms can be due to hypothyroidism so it may be worth getting checked, especially if you feel sluggish and fatigued. I don't. I actually feel full of energy and my thyroid is normal. The symptoms are the result of losing a great deal of weight.

Exercise is one way to get those metabolic processes going. The other way is to eat more protein, which makes the metabolism produce heat-generating reactions. Maybe I'll always be cold – some people are. I have spoken to others who have lost substantial amounts of weight and found that they are cold too.

The thing to do is to persuade your body to switch from 'conserve' to 'burn' mode. The only ways to do this are to increase protein intake and to exercise more.

So just keep moving. I can't offer more than that and it isn't easy when you work at a desk, though it helps to take frequent breaks and dash up and down stairs a few times. It is extremely unpleasant being very cold but I'll accept it as one of the prices to pay for a substantial weight loss. Unfortunately the body's thermostat does not seem to return to normal unless you put some weight back.

The most important thing to keep in mind if you encounter weight-loss difficulties is that there is always a way through, over or round them. But it's also important to know that there may be a time to stop losing for a while and maintain, increasing your calorie intake by just enough to do so. A long run of apparently insuperable difficulties may be your body's way of saying enough. For now, at any rate.

Chapter Twelve
Keeping It Off For Ever

How Much Weight Should You Lose?

This is a quote from a doctor in a book about weight loss:[1]

> It is my honest belief that the vast majority of individuals instinctively know what is a good weight for them, and that this is a relatively personal and individual issue...an individual's sense of his or her ideal weight or size really is the most appropriate target to aim for.

But don't get excited, he doesn't mean it. The book contains the usual dire warnings about weight and health along with those awful BMI charts, and – yawn – I'm still obese. Perplexingly, the doctor says that one of the problems of the BMI chart is its broad band of 'healthy weight'. A woman of 5′ 6″, he says, could be between 8 st 2 lb and 10 st 4 lb and still be in the healthy band. So? What is your point, doctor? (He says his point is that the healthy band is too wide to give an individual an idea of their ideal weight. I say the whole BMI chart fails to give an individual an idea of their ideal weight.)

So let's have a quote from another doctor, the Australian Rick Kausman, in *his* book about weight loss:[2]

> What is a healthy weight for an individual can only be determined by that particular person looking after themselves in the healthiest way they can, living in the environment of the day. As a result of doing that, their weight will evolve to the healthiest level that is possible.

Kausman, like me, rejects BMI charts and height/weight tables because 'the so-called ideal weights are set at levels that are far too low. The weights are not representative of the current population, let alone applicable to an individual.'[3]

When you are very heavy it is difficult not to have a 'target weight' in your mind. There are pitfalls, as Kausman points out: you might not reach it, you might not maintain it. I think it has to be an individual choice. When I started losing weight I certainly didn't set my target at 13 stone. The idea of losing six and a half stone would have been inconceivable – it's a whole person (someone of 'ideal weight' on the bloody BMI chart!) No, if I'd walked in to that Slimming World class thinking, here I am at nearly 20 stone and what I'd really like to be is 13, I'd have walked right out again. I would not have believed it possible.

So if you must have a target weight make it a realistic one and get there in small stages. My own opinion, unpopular though this may be, is that if you have been very large for a number of years, then planning to reach nine stone or less is probably not realistic. Jill Welbourne agrees, adding that if you have been very heavy, you will actually not feel comfortable in your body at a much lower weight. You will feel unbalanced. If you are used to carrying an 18-stone body an eight-stone one will not feel right. Your centre of gravity will have shifted. And the same principles explored in Chapter 9 apply here: you do not have to get down to any particular weight any more than you have to lose it in the first place.

Besides, a very practical and important consideration is that the lower you go, the fewer calories your body will require and the more likely you are to be hungry. At eight stone your basic calorie requirement (the amount you'd need in a coma) would be from 1037 to 1240. Obviously you can eat more as soon as you get up from the bed but you won't have a great deal of leeway.

Professor Philip James of the International Obesity Task Force has admitted that 'It's a tragedy that we in the medical profession, backed up by streams of articles, have this idea of a goal weight. It's a recipe for generating people who are constantly in agony.'[4]

What about all the horrendous health risks of great weight, you might ask? Well, if you need a statistic at all, go by this one: 'When an overweight person loses even 10 per cent of body weight and keeps it off, most adverse medical consequences of excess fat subside, whether or not the loss brings the person into some predetermined weight bracket.'[5] If you bring exercise into the equation, any health risks you *may* have from excess weight are also substantially reduced.

Why Do so Many Gain the Weight Back?

1. They don't eat enough on their diet. Most dieters fall into this trap because they follow 'the X diet' (diets with names never work long term) or they set themselves a too-restricted, daily calorie allowance. You cannot maintain a diet of less than 1400 calories per day. You can stay on a lower calorie intake for a while, but not for ever. Even if you exercise gargantuan amounts of will power for a long period, your body will *make* you eat more in the end. Every single low-calorie diet ends in weight regain.

2. They lose weight too fast, either through a diet too low in energy or a fitness regime that cannot be maintained for life. Very often people combine the two, which results in a very fast weight loss, a feeling of physical achievement and toned-ness and the exultant sense of having cracked it. Then they find they can keep up neither the diet nor the punishing regime in the gym and back comes the weight.

3. When they hit a plateau they panic. They reduce calorie intake drastically. See point 1 above.

4. Or they get despondent when they reach a plateau. The diet doesn't seem to be working, so they give up.

5. They include exercise as part of the weight-loss plan but after a while they decrease the exercise (energy output) without downwardly adjusting their calorie intake.

6. They reach a weight that is acceptable to them, finish the diet and go back to 'normal' eating. Even if 'normal' pre-diet eating was only 2000 calories a day, the recommended intake for the average women, the dieting mechanism means that the body will have become far more efficient at storing calories and the metabolic requirement will have fallen with the weight loss. If weight was previously maintained on 2000 calories, now it will be gained on that amount, even if the weight was lost slowly; you will still have a dieted body, crying out to restore itself.

7. They have an emotional problem with eating which the diet has not addressed. When stress, grief or depression occurs they

cannot help turning to food. This has nothing to do with will power or weakness. It is such an essential factor in weight fluctuation that anyone who sees their eating being sabotaged in this way really does need professional counselling or therapy. If they can't afford it they should put immense pressure on their GP. After all, it is the medical profession who puts pressure on us to lose weight; it is their responsibility to provide the help that is needed.

8. For reasons that may be complex and not immediately accessible, they may not want to be thinner. Loss of weight can be unconsciously associated with loss of power. However compelling the social or aesthetic reasons for wanting to lose weight, if fatness is serving a purpose it will return. I have mentioned women like Sheila Kitzinger and Jill Welbourne, who are very aware that they need their weight for power and presence. Others, perhaps not so aware, may find that only when they are large are they taken seriously: this can apply to women doing traditional 'men's work'. Or there may be a history of sexual abuse; it is very very common for an abused person to become fat to protect themselves. When they lose weight, they lose that sense of protection. Because so much of this is unconscious, good counselling is essential.

9. They aim for an unrealistically low weight. Unrealistic can be 10 stone for a woman who starts at 20 stone or even 16 stone. Either she cannot cope with the long haul, or she cannot maintain the new weight because it is too low and so is the calorie intake required to sustain it.

How to Keep the Weight Off

What is more important than the amount of weight you lose is the way your body reacts to the loss. As I hope I have shown, even very slow weight loss causes the body to go into a state of alarm. The more weight you lose the less you will be able to eat, for two reasons: the lighter body requires fewer calories, and your system will be in conserve mode.

You need to be very attentive to your body's cries. When plateaus become longer and longer it's time to think about stopping. Even if at some later date you decide to try and shed more weight, a prolonged period of stasis on a diet indicates that right now your body wants you to have a break from dieting. All these things will vary according to your age, your weight and your previous dieting history. The lengthening plateau phases are a warning. Jill Welbourne recommends pursuing active weight loss in the summer, May to December, then allowing yourself to plateau from December to May. It is always more difficult to lose weight in the winter because the body's alarm system is on red alert: you've lost tissue and you need it because it's cold.

My intention is to remain at 13 stone. My present resting metabolic rate (RMR) is 1532 calories. In ten years time, if I am the same weight, it will have dropped to 1350. You can raise this by increasing exercise but you have to keep in mind that you will have to be able to sustain this. Stopping exercise is like stopping dieting: the result is rebound weight gain.

If you diet from, say, 15 to 9 stone and you are aged between 30 and 59 your resting metabolic rate (RMR) will fall from 1639 to 1323. When you are 60 or over it will be 1116 or over. That's a big drop in intake. The more you lose the less you will be able to eat; the less you can eat the more likely you are to put the weight back on. I find a RMR of about 1500 something I can live with. That's what you have to calculate in deciding when to stop dieting.

When you finish the active part of losing weight, you face maintenance. And I'm sorry, all you who are anti-diet, but this is danger time. The keyword here is vigilance. You don't have to count calories all the time, though a food diary is still useful to monitor trends. And though many disagree, I recommend a decent set of scales (I don't actually see what is so terrible about weighing yourself). Get something that you can trust for accuracy, like the German make Soehnle, which are a bit more pricey but worth it. The cheaper scales can both under- and over-weigh and can be irritatingly inconsistent. The thing about weighing yourself is that you won't then put on a stone without knowing it – and it's easy to do that if you have a dieted body.

Do not weigh more than once a week. You'll probably want to do this for the first few weeks because you won't really believe that you can hold your new weight. When you've been very heavy and then spent a long time slowly losing it, the idea of actually maintaining a new lower weight can feel alien and a bit scary. You are convinced at first that it's all going to come piling back on. When you are happy that you can maintain, weigh yourself about once a fortnight.

Don't keep the scales in the kitchen or bathroom. Keep them somewhere you would not normally go, like a spare bedroom, rather than a room you are in several times a day. This is because people who have lost weight invariably feel anxious about putting it on again and if the scales are too accessible you'll be hopping on and off all day or every day. Mine are in the hall by the front door. We never, ever use the front door (for all we know there could be corpses piled up outside it: people who 'came and no one answered'!), so we never go into the hall.

You need to experiment with your diet. You need to find a way of eating that satisfies you and which will keep your weight stable. Eat what you want but, until you get accustomed to what works, keep counting in some form or other. Keep fat intake to around 30 per cent of total calories. And you need to keep up your levels of activity. I hope by now that 'gym' will be a dirty word in your fitness lexicon, and that you will simply be whizzing all over the place and up and down stairs. Even if you are disabled, there are simple, calorie-burning exercises you can try to work into your daily routine.

It may be that you gain a couple of pounds before you stabilise. If you do, don't respond to this by dieting. Just keep an eye on it. You will not be able to forget about your new weight; for the dieter, maintaining a stable weight is very different from the non-dieter doing so. My husband never watches what he eats and would never weigh himself. Sometimes I ask him to out of interest (mine, not his!). Whatever he eats, however many feasts and holidays and eating splurges he indulges in, his weight stays the same, within two or three pounds. But then he has never dieted.

Remember that your body has marshalled its forces and would like to help you regain what you have lost. The old bod is a bit bewildered by all this; throughout its life you've fed it, overfed it and starved it, probably with no sort of consistency or regularity. Now there's been a period of famine, albeit a mild one, and it's ready to fill the grain stores. Just think of all those empty, billowing little adipocytes and that panic-buying enzyme, lipoprotein lipase, looking for fat to lay down in store, and the metabolism, ticking away slowly so that it can conserve with greater efficiency.

You must feed your body well. But you can never abandon the diet. Work out your resting metabolic rate, gauge your calorie requirements from the chart in the Appendix, keep exercising and don't let things slide. I have been amazed at how much eating has to do with habit and how easy it would be to slip back into old patterns, especially if you are living with other people who eat in an ad hoc kind of way and don't have to count or monitor their intake. It would be easy to join them. And it's fine to do so occasionally.

Arabella Churchill, granddaughter of the great Winston, has inherited his looks and tendency to portliness. Her life is nothing if not adventurous and when she was shipwrecked in the late nineties, she decided, as she clung all night to the wreckage, that if she survived she would make some changes.

Not one to do anything by halves she decided to have a face lift – performed live on the internet. Newspapers were full of the forthcoming event, but Arabella had been ordered by her surgeon to lose three stone before the operation.

She went to Weight Watchers, where she reduced her weight from 15 st 2 lbs to 12 st 2 lbs. So delighted was she with the way she looked she decided she did not want the face lift after all. Full of energy and determination she resolved to keep the weight off.

About a year later she had put back two of the three stone. At the time of writing she has lost weight again and is now $12\frac{1}{2}$ stone. So what went wrong?

'Travelling round the world a lot, not being careful about what I was eating, not having access to a weighing machine or a full-length mirror,' she says. 'And generally just becoming slack about it.'

There is is in a nutshell. Stop the diet and the weight comes back.

You can keep the weight off, but you don't have to take my word for it. An interesting study has shown what I've long suspected – that it really is possible. The largest ever study of dieters who had maintained their weight loss long term (five years) was carried out at the University of Pittsburgh School of Medicine in conjunction with the University of Colorado Health Sciences Center. A total of 784 very overweight people (629 of them women) lost an average of 29 per cent of their body weight (66 lbs). The minimum weight reduction maintained was 30 lbs.

Most of the participants (73 per cent) had a family history of fatness, with at least one overweight parent, and all were considerably overweight. By the age of 18, most had become large. Most said that they were more committed to losing weight permanently than in previous attempts, a significant finding. Half-hearted attempts are always doomed to failure; readiness, commitment and singlemindedness are the key.

To maintain their weight loss, 92 per cent of the participants limited their consumption of certain kinds of foods; almost 50 per cent reported restricting the quantity of food consumed; 38 per cent reduced the percentage of fat calories consumed; 35.5 per cent counted calories; and 30 per cent counted fat grams. Many reported restricting their fat intake to 24 per cent of total calories, preparing most of their meals at home. About 90 per cent changed both their eating and their exercise patterns.

The overwhelming majority of the group reported dramatic improvements in their personal and professional lives. Over 85 per cent reported feeling more energetic, self-confident, healthier and in a better mood than before losing the weight. More than half reported improved job performance as well as bettter relationships with friends and others.[6] While the improvements may have been the result of simply taking positive action of *some* kind, there is no doubt that weight loss does lead to greater confidence, success and achievement in many areas of life.[7]

Not everyone loses weight in the same way at the same rate. Similarly, not everyone maintains their weight loss using the same method. In the end though there is one common factor: those who achieve long-term weight loss keep their average daily calorie intake lower than it was when they were large. They may also work on their energy expenditure: exercise.

There may always be an underlying anxiety about regaining the weight you have lost but I think that is no bad thing. While you can and should eat with enjoyment, complacency waits around the corner and complacency is the death knell of the successful diet.

It is essential to remember that for those of us who have become very large, food has played a part far beyond its remit. We have used it for more than fuel: food has been a huge part of our social and emotional life. In the end it became too important.

Food is never the enemy. I love food now more than ever – perhaps *because* it is rationed. What I have to remember is that I cannot relax and eat like other people – at least, not for more than one day at a time. The proof that once you lose weight you cannot return to normal eating resides in my own body. I am dieting – in that I am counting and cutting back to make up for those days where I *do* eat like everyone else – and my weight is now stable. I am dieting without losing weight.

The temptation after a diet is to start having 'normal' days one after the other. Unless your diet has left you with a particularly small appetite, you can't do that.

The other night I woke at 3.30 a.m. feeling anxious about my weight. In a half-sleep I got up, went downstairs to the hall and weighed myself. It was okay.

Poor sad cow, you might think. Maybe. But considering I am a happier, fitter person, being a 'sad cow' is fine by me. Eternal vigilance does not seem too high a price to pay.

The next chapter contains the stories of five women who lost weight and kept it off – some for over 20 years. They all had different methods; they all found what suited them best.

Good luck.

Chapter Thirteen
How They Did It: Stories from the Five per Cent

In searching for real-life stories of those who had lost weight and maintained the loss, I found the 95 per cent figure borne out. So of the 100 or so people I canvassed, here are the five. Their methods of losing weight vary a great deal; their maintenance is also different and in some cases, idiosyncratic, but weight loss is never a one-size-fits-all matter.

Judith Durham

Judith Durham shot to stardom in the sixties as the beautiful lead singer of the Australian group The Seekers, who at the height of their fame were bigger than the Beatles and the Rolling Stones. Though success followed success, though men fell in love with her and women wanted to emulate her, Judith was deeply unhappy about her weight.

She had begun to comfort eat as a teenager and as time went by she found it more and more difficult to deal with stress without eating. Drinking coffee to try to suppress her appetite only seemed to make her hungrier. Food never seemed satisfying enough. 'Everyone always called it puppy fat which used to upset me because I knew I had a major eating problem,' she says.

Judith was completely unprepared for The Seekers' success with their first record, 'I'll Never Find Another You'. Weighing just under 11 stone and only 5′ 2″ she panicked and tried to lose weight.

I dressed carefully so as not to look my weight – always pulled my waist in and wore high heels, a lot of dark colours and dresses that hugged my ribs over waistlength bras and elastic girdles. I really started to lose weight at the time 'I'll Never Find Another You' was going up the charts. But I still would have been 10 stone on the day we reached Number 1 for the first time.

Twiggy became major news a year after that, and there was even more pressure to look hip and cool in the Carnaby Street image à la Sandie Shaw or Cilla Black. At that time, I felt more and more pressure to try to look the part of the pop star. It never occurred to me to accept myself as I was or realise that other people really liked me. I didn't like myself like that. I wanted to be the glamour queen. I didn't realise that even Marilyn Monroe was heavy by those standards. I loathed my body image – I always believed that I wasn't meant to look like that. And I still believe that in a way. I didn't like my face and thought it was very fat – which it was. I couldn't see the beauty that others apparently saw in it. I wanted to have plastic surgery. It came as a shock when my husband-to-be said 'What a dolly lady' when he first met me – I didn't realise such a transformation had taken place. About 10 years after, the photographer who shot the cover of the 'Hot Jazz Duo' album said that I was 'pretty' and I nearly died of shock then, too.

Like most people desperate to lose weight, Judith had made countless attempts using different diets. 'I had a yo-yo diet history. I tried every diet under the sun. I was an expert at lots of crash diets and exercise fads. My mother couldn't take me seriously when I announced that I was going to be a vegetarian for the rest of my life (which I will be!).'

In 1969, Judith married Ron Edgeworth, a brilliant pianist, and he introduced her to a spiritual path that included vegetarianism. Plagued since early childhood with bronchiectasis, a progressive lung condition with no cure (the worst thing a singer could have), Judith then found a diet that seemed miraculous. It helped clear the mucus which constantly built up in her lungs and she lost weight.

It was the Professor Arnold Ehret books that gave me answers. I found I could eat so much more food, and the foods didn't create that same kind of hunger. It is fruit and low-carbohydrate vegetables and olive oil – and very little protein or carbohydrate. I have soya milk these days, but of course when I first embraced the diet there was no soya milk around in the shops at all. That is a luxury I allow myself now and I think I benefit from it. Hope so.

Sometimes I crave protein and carbohydrate foods, but these cravings have become less and less. I feel best when I am on only fruit or during the mornings before I have even eaten anything at all, after only a cup of decaf tea and soya milk for instance, or after an early glass of grape juice.

Before Ehret, when I was still eating meat, I lost weight by cutting out fancy foods. For instance, I wouldn't eat bread or biscuits or ice cream. I even had lamb chops for breakfast so that I wouldn't eat toast. I lost my first stone during that time. At the time I met Ron I was already down to about $8\frac{1}{2}$ stone. I think that's why he was attracted to me. Once I undertook the natural lifestyle Ron was already starting to follow, I lost more weight, mainly because of spasmodic fasting and juice and fruit and vegetable regimes.

I don't think people realise what an amazing thing this is for me. People tend to almost ridicule me when I tell them I had a major problem in that area. I believe that by now I could have been dead if I had carried on the way I was going in the early sixties, or certainly I would be carrying an enormous amount of weight. Once I found the Arnold Ehret diet, I can say that my major problems with food were over. At last I could freely eat large quantities of food. I did have cravings and binged occasionally, but I always had my safety net of the diet that I knew was my foundation. I would not like to say that I am at my 'desired' weight now – I think I am actually too thin – but I no longer have an overweight problem, which is a much happier state for me to be in. I think my best weight would actually be about half a stone heavier, but I have to eat lightly because of my lung capacity. It is an automatic process; I have a cut-off capacity for food beyond which I simply cannot physically eat more, or I get too breathless.

The main reason for me to stick to the diet so stringently now is that it helps my breathing; the bronchiectasis I contracted at the age of four after measles has gradually worsened, and is now quite severe. This was one of the main reasons I undertook the Arnold Ehret diet in the first place; hoping it would free me of mucus problems. However, the side-effect of the diet is that it seems to keep my weight constant.

I don't think I would ever want to put on weight now – not while I'm in the public eye and trying to sing. To be honest, I would fear it, because I have to be very strict with my diet in order to have enough breath. I find the diet helps my breathing a great deal, and I stick rigidly to a fairly spartan diet when I am on a concert tour. So it will be interesting to see what happens when I retire. I think I would get too breathless to be comfortable and enjoy life if I ate the typical vegetarian diet I used to eat. I used to eat lots of rice, nuts, bread, etc, which are foods I actually now avoid. It's just too much food for me now.

Judith's diet is unconventional and many would frown on it. But I know Judith Durham and there is no denying the beneficial effect on her that this diet has had. Apart from the fact that she has maintained her weight loss for over 20 years, her voice is better and richer than ever; logically, with her lung disease worsening all the time (she only has 40 per cent capacity) this should not be so. Judith is the first to recognise that her diet would not suit everyone.

I am wary of recommending the diet I am on to others. That it is the lesser of many evils is all I can say. I have a lot of health problems – skin problems, osteoporosis, shocking lung problems and high blood pressure among them. But I have enormous energy and I am rarely acutely ill. I do not seem to get the flu or infections like so many others and I don't seem to tire or get depressed. I would say I handle stress well.

I believe that people need to try to lose weight for the right motives; ie for health and energy and economy of food. I think we need to eat every morsel with gratitude and care and attention to what we are actually doing – which is taking of life, even if it is a humble carrot that is being sacrificed for our needs. I think we should always be aware of why we are eating at any time. Even if we are eating to de-stress I think we need to acknowledge that motive, so that we don't eat with any guilt or shame – ever. Eating is a wonderful gift.

Esther Rantzen

It's hard to imagine the tiny, blonde broadcaster Esther Rantzen as a hefty brunette but that is what she was for many years. Though a thin child, she followed the pattern of her mother and aunts and put on weight when she was 16.

I'm sure it was hormones that made me eat. It was definitely comfort eating. Whether it was related to sex I don't know. I was quite a late developer. I was 16 in 1956, around the time that Marilyn Monroe was the sex goddess and everyone was so thrilled with the idea of her being a size 16. She was curvy. I was curvy but with the wrong sorts of curves. I went in where I should go out and out where I should go in. It was horrible, I was just too heavy – a couple of stone overweight, which on someone my height is quite a lot.

Although I was eating a lot, I didn't enjoy it. The food went down so fast, I didn't even chew it. I seemed to have some sort of void and sweet food was what I needed. I thought that being fat was the problem in my life and if I got thin everything would be okay.

I was totally self-conscious about my weight at university. I did have boyfriends but I felt it incumbent upon me to be entertaining for them. This often happens with overweight; look at the number of performers with weight problems. I went through university much too fat. I tried every diet there was and they were all revolting.

When I went to work for the BBC, I was happy and occupied and I didn't need to eat for comfort any more. The weight fell off. But it hasn't always been plain sailing. I gave up smoking and put on weight. I took up smoking again because I was so petrified of getting fat again, but I did finally give up for good.

Esther believes that she has kept the weight off by eating good plain home-cooked food and not very much of it.

A meal is not a treat for me. I think it was all those horrible diets I did – they put me off food! I can sit in a restaurant and not want anything on the menu but if you gave me a fresh new-laid egg with soldiers – well, that's different. In a restaurant, I'll scrape sauces off, or remove things from their pastry. I love ordinary day-to-day food. I eat by appetite. Sometimes I'll wake up ravenously hungry and realise it's because I didn't have supper the night before. If I have one big meal a day I don't get hungry.

Jackie Ballard

Jackie Ballard, former MP for Taunton, also found that being in the public eye made her self-conscious about her high weight. Though she wished it were not so, she felt the pressure to lose weight was too great for her to resist.

I've been dieting for as far back as I can remember. I did all those teenage diets – you know, an apple and a celery stick – and the diet would last about a week. I don't remember a time when I wasn't dieting or thinking about my weight. I went to Weight Watchers a couple of times and loathed it. The only time I lost weight was when I was pregnant – and then I was actually told to eat more for the first time in my life! I put weight on after having the baby but didn't make much attempt to lose it. I toyed with the occasional diet but nothing serious.

Then a few years ago, a good friend, who had always been about my size, lost six or seven stone. She'd always seemed very comfortable with her weight and dressed confidently, not going around in baggy dark clothes like I did. I used to think, why can't I be more like her instead of trying to hide my body? When I asked her why she'd lost weight she just said 'I don't want to be fat for the rest of my life.' I decided the same was true for me.

There were motivating factors in my life. After my divorce, my weight had been a defence mechanism: if I was fat I would not be sexually desirable and therefore not available. I didn't want anyone to come near me. Three years ago I became conscious of what those emotional blocks were and realised that the issue was not about my weight, it was about not wanting a relationship; not wanting to risk being sexually desirable. And I decided that perhaps I did want a relationship.

Then Auberon Waugh – who used to say vitriolic things about me in his column – wrote that he didn't see how I could be an MP since I was too fat to get through the voting lobby. That really hurt.

I had a health scare, too; at the time it seemed it was a heart problem, though it turned out not to be. It made me aware that I didn't want to run that risk, especially as I knew that the menopause was likely to make me put on more weight.

So I asked my friend how to do it. We decided I'd wait until the beginning of August when Parliament finished. I went to a health farm for four days to detox, then I went to stay with my friend. I went to the gym with her and she helped me kickstart the diet. I lost five stone in a year. I can be very disciplined.

I did have some letters from women in the Party saying that they felt I'd sold out. I'd made a virtue of being liberal, and saying that we should be allowed to be anything we want without being discriminated against, so they felt I was being a traitor. But it's harder for women to be overweight. Nicholas Soames and John Prescott can get away with it; Ann Widdecombe can't.

I realise that sexual attractiveness is not about weight *per se*, it's how you feel about yourself. Of course you can be very big and sexy – look at Dawn French. But it's only when you can feel good about yourself that you transmit that sort of glow, and that's how I felt after I lost weight.

I've relaxed a bit and started eating some of the things I'd given up. I put 5 lbs on over New Year but managed to lose it within a fornight. I want to go back on the diet and lose another 2 stone but I'm finding it difficult to get back into it. I do weigh myself twice a week and I plot it on a graph. There is a line above which I will not allow myself to go; it's an arbitrary line chosen by me but it's a psychological thing. I am confident I will not put the weight back on again.

Jackie's diet is sound and she does not allow herself to get hungry.

A Typical Day
Breakfast: Branflakes with fruit juice, banana.

Lunch: Tuna or salmon with salad, no dressing.

Dinner: Hot meal – fish with cooked vegetables.

During the day I eat as much fruit as I like; I can eat a pound of grapes at a time. I never feel hungry. I don't drink alcohol, I drink mineral water. If I have a meal out I have fish and salad and fresh fruit to follow. And I don't count calories.

Alice Marchant

But you do not have to be in the public eye to lose weight successfully. Alice was 40 when she decided that a history of yo-yo dieting and accumulated weight from three pregnancies was going to be a thing of the past once and for all.

I'd been fat since I was about 14 but living up north it didn't seem to matter so much. Northern women are not as neurotic about their weight as southerners! I was just a good, strapping, healthy girl. But I was a size 14 and that's quite big for someone in their early teens.

I dieted for my wedding; I was about 12 stone by then. I looked lovely on The Day in a size-12 dress and thought that was it, I'd stay that weight for ever. I'd counted calories very strictly: 900 some days, 1100 on others and 1300 at weekends. It really didn't seem too difficult. I decided that when I finished the diet I'd just try and eat very sensibly. I did, I ate loads of low-fat stuff, but the weight crept back. Then I was pregnant and starving; I put on four stone. I was 15 stone when I gave birth.

To cut a long story a bit shorter, I weighed 17 stone after my third child was born and by then I'd tried a good few diets. They all worked – diets do – but I could never keep them going and the weight came back plus a lot more. Anyway, after Helen was born, I was breastfeeding and I thought that meant you could eat what you liked because all the calories were used up making milk. What a doddle, I thought. But be warned, girls, it isn't quite like that. When I weaned her I weighed 18 stone. And my fortieth birthday was approaching.

I was miserable. I couldn't move easily, my back hurt and I couldn't look in a mirror. The children were teased at school because of their fat mum and my heart broke for them. I knew I couldn't afford to try another diet that would let me down so I joined a slimming club.

That was ten years ago. What can I say except that it worked? I lost seven stone in three years. I think what made it work was a realistic eating plan and the support of other people, including my family. What *kept* it working was that I never actually stopped dieting. I'd seen that my pattern had always been diet – lose weight – stop dieting – gain weight – and that had recurred many, many times. This time, when I'd reached my target weight of 11 stone I stayed on the diet. I do eat more than I did when I was losing but I watch it all the time. I weigh myself every Saturday morning in my nightie and if my weight goes up I cut back a little. After holidays I go straight back on the club's plan for a couple of weeks because I don't think you can help putting on weight on holiday. I don't beat myself up about it, I just accept that it's going to happen. I usually put on about half a stone.

My own experience tells me that you can't ever stop dieting once you've got the weight off. Once you accept that it's for life, it's not too difficult. I'd rather that than the depression of having gained loads of weight yet again so I'm quite happy. I do have treats, chocolate and cakes, sometimes but I just allow for them. I wouldn't have it any other way.

Meriel Chambers

Meriel is a 38-year-old university research fellow who had a compulsive eating disorder in her teens and twenties.

By the time I was 25 and working for my PhD I weighed 20 stone. I got a reputation for being a standoffish academic and indeed I had very little to do with my colleagues but this was not because I was unfriendly. I could not bear being seen. I would stay in my room as much as possible. And I just grew bigger and bigger.

I ate gargantuan amounts. I would have a meal with three or four thick slices of bread and butter. I'd have a large pudding. I could eat a whole cheesecake. There were certain foods I could *only* eat compulsively and in large quantities and I didn't seem to have the emotional stamina to avoid them. I'd buy a box of eclairs and eat the lot. If I didn't have something to eat I'd panic. I tried so hard to bring it under control but I seemed to have no free will about it. I'd make myself try to limit my intake but then I'd break out and go and buy a huge bar of chocolate.

It was such a shameful thing, like a dirty little secret but a secret that I couldn't hide because I was wearing it. When I reached 20 stone I went to a counsellor in absolute desperation. I don't much believe in psychology – it's too inexact a science for me – but I have to admit it helped. The counsellor looked at some issues in my past and although I couldn't see any direct connection, I did the work conscientiously.

Eight years ago I felt ready to tackle my eating. I did it strictly scientifically, by counting calories. I aimed for a slow weight loss of about a pound a week. At first it came off much more quickly than that but I knew it would slow down. In every other way I had been a fairly disciplined sort of person and so the maths involved in this method appealed to me. I eat about 1600 calories now and my weight has been stable at 14 stone for five years. I actually enjoy dieting. I love the way I feel; 14 stone is not what I'd choose but, believe me, when you've been 20 it feels sylph-like! I'd like to lose more but I'm afraid that if I cut my calorie intake further I'll be hungry and the compulsive behaviour might start again. For my height of 5′ 8″ 14 stone is not too bad. I know I'll always have to count calories – it's about science – but it can be very satisfying knowing that by doing so I'm not going to be hugely fat again.

What all these women have found is that permanent weight loss means a diet for life. Even Esther Rantzen, though no longer consciously dieting, chooses her food so that her overall calorie intake keeps her on maintenance. All admit to the occasional binge; dieting does not mean you have to lose your humanity! In this respect the parallel with alcoholism and other addictions is slightly more tenuous; it is a lot easier to get back onto the dieting path than the non-drinking, smoking or drug-taking one.

Keeping the weight off requires mindfulness. It does not need obsessive thinking about food but an awareness of what we are doing: eating, as Judith Durham says, 'with care and attention'.

There will be times when you come adrift. Your emotions and life events will make it more difficult at times to eat with that care and attention. You may gain some weight. Maintaining weight loss does not mean you *never* gain any.

If I've had a few days away or a run of celebratory meals I enjoy them, put on a few pounds and then get back to the diet. As Judith says, the diet can be your 'safety net'. If you can't cope with restricted eating at difficult times, try at least to eat as closely as possible to your own particular weight-loss plan.

That's the essence of long-term maintenance: not losing sight of the way you lost the weight.

And will I keep the weight off? I believe so, this time. For the first time in my dieting history the end fully justify the means.

Appendix
Basal Metabolic Rate[1]

Daily energy (kilocalorie) requirements of women aged 18–29 years

Body Weight (Stones)	Basal Metabolic Rate	Total energy requirement (kcal per day)		
		Sedentary	Active	Very Active
7	1146	1720	1950	2180
7.5	1193	1790	2030	2270
8	1240	1860	2110	2360
8.5	1288	1930	2190	2450
9	1335	2000	2270	2540
9.5	1382	2070	2350	2630
10	1428	2140	2430	2710
10.5	1476	2210	2510	2800
11	1523	2280	2590	2890
11.5	1570	2360	2670	2980
12	1618	2430	2750	3070
12.5	1664	2500	2830	3160
13	1711	2570	2910	3250
13.5	1758	2640	2990	3340
14	1806	2710	3070	3430
14.5	1853	2780	3150	3520
15	1900	2850	3230	3610
15.5	1945	2918	3306	3696
16	1992	2988	3386	3785
16.5	2040	3060	3468	3876
17	2087	3130	3548	3965
17.5	2133	3200	3628	4053
18	2180	3270	3706	4142
18.5	2228	3342	3788	4233
19	2274	3411	3866	4321
19.5	2320	3480	3944	4408
20	2370	3555	4029	4503

For every additional stone increase daily calorie intake by 100

Daily energy (kilocalorie) requirements of women aged 30–59 years

Body Weight (Stones)	Basal Metabolic Rate	Total energy requirement (kcal per day)		
		Sedentary	Active	Very Active
7	1215	1820	2070	2310
7.5	1242	1860	2110	2360
8	1268	1900	2160	2410
8.5	1295	1940	2190	2450
9	1323	1980	2250	2510
9.5	1348	2020	2290	2560
10	1374	2060	2340	2610
10.5	1400	2100	2380	2660
11	1427	2140	2430	2710
11.5	1454	2180	2470	2760
12	1480	2220	2520	2810
12.5	1505	2260	2560	2860
13	1532	2300	2600	2910
13.5	1559	2340	2650	2960
14	1586	2380	2700	3010
14.5	1612	2420	2740	3060
15	1639	2460	2790	3110
15.5	1645	2468	2796	3126
16	1671	2506	2841	3175
16.5	1700	2550	2890	3230
17	1723	2584	2929	3274
17.5	1750	2625	2975	3325
18	1774	2661	3016	3371
18.5	1800	2700	3060	3420
19	1825	2738	3102	3468
19.5	1852	2778	3148	3519
20	1880	2820	3196	3572

For every additional stone increase daily calorie intake by 50

Appendix

Daily energy (kilocalorie) requirements of women aged 60 years and over

Body Weight (Stones)	Basal Metabolic Rate	Total energy requirement (kcal per day)		
		Sedentary	Active	Very Active
7	998	1500	1700	1900
7.5	1028	1542	1750	1950
8	1057	1590	1800	2010
8.5	1087	1630	1850	2070
9	1116	1670	1900	2120
9.5	1146	1720	1950	2180
10	1174	1760	2000	2230
10.5	1204	1810	2050	2290
11	1233	1850	2100	2340
11.5	1263	1890	2150	2400
12	1292	1940	2200	2450
12.5	1320	1980	2250	2510
13	1350	2030	2300	2570
13.5	1380	2070	2350	2620
14	1409	2110	2400	2680
14.5	1439	2160	2450	2730
15	1469	2200	2500	2790
15.5	1552	2298	2590	2907
16	1581	2327	2688	3004
16.5	1610	2415	2737	3059
17	1639	2458	2786	3114
17.5	1667	2500	2834	3167
18	1697	2546	2885	3224
18.5	1726	2589	2934	3279
19	1754	2631	2982	3333
19.5	1783	2674	3031	3388
20	1810	2715	3077	3439

For every additional stone increase daily calorie intake by 50

Daily energy (kilocalorie) requirements of men aged 18–29 years

Body Weight (Stones)	Basal Metabolic Rate	Total energy requirement (kcal per day)		
		Sedentary	Active	Very Active
8	1456	2180	2480	2770
8.5	1509	2260	2570	2870
9	1557	2340	2650	2960
9.5	1606	2140	2730	3050
10	1652	2480	2810	3140
10.5	1701	2550	2890	3230
11	1749	2620	2970	3320
11.5	1797	2700	3060	3410
12	1846	2770	3410	3510
12.5	1892	2840	3220	3600
13	1940	2910	3300	3690
13.5	1990	2980	3380	3780
14	2037	3060	3460	3870
14.5	2086	3130	3550	3960
15	2134	3200	3630	4050
15.5	2180	3270	3710	4140
16	2220	3330	3770	4220
16.5	2278	3420	3870	4330
17	2330	3490	3950	4420
17.5	2365	3548	4020	4494
18	2410	3615	4097	4579
18.5	2460	3690	4182	4674
19	2510	3765	4267	4769
19.5	2555	3832	4344	4854
20	2605	3908	4428	4950

For every additional stone increase daily calorie intake by 100

Daily energy (kilocalorie) requirements of men aged 30–59 years

Body Weight (Stones)	Basal Metabolic Rate	Total energy requirement (kcal per day)		
		Sedentary	Active	Very Active
8	1458	2190	2480	2770
8.5	1495	2240	2540	2840
9	1532	2300	2600	2910
9.5	1569	2350	2670	2980
10	1604	2410	2730	3050
10.5	1641	2460	2790	3120
11	1678	2520	2850	3190
11.5	1715	2570	2920	3260
12	1752	2630	2980	3330
12.5	1787	2680	3040	3400
13	1824	2740	3100	3470
13.5	1861	2790	3160	3540
14	1898	2850	3230	3610
14.5	1934	2900	3290	3680
15	1970	2960	3350	3750
15.5	2007	3010	3410	3810
16	2037	3060	3460	3870
16.5	2080	3120	3540	3950
17	2117	3180	3600	4020
17.5	2150	3225	3655	4085
18	2184	3276	3713	4150
18.5	2220	3330	3774	4218
19	2260	3390	3842	4294
19.5	2295	3442	3902	4360
20	2330	3495	3961	4427

For every additional stone increase daily calorie intake by 50

Daily energy (kilocalorie) requirements of men aged 60 years and over

Body Weight (Stones)	Basal Metabolic Rate	Total energy requirement (kcal per day)		
		Sedentary	Active	Very Active
8	1182	1773	2009	2246
8.5	1220	1830	2074	2318
9	1256	1884	2135	2386
9.5	1294	1941	2200	2459
10	1331	1996	2263	2529
10.5	1368	2052	2326	2599
11	1406	2109	2390	2671
11.5	1443	2164	2453	2742
12	1480	2220	2516	2812
12.5	1517	2276	2579	2882
13	1555	2332	2644	2954
13.5	1591	2386	2705	3023
14	1629	2444	2769	3095
14.5	1666	2499	2832	3165
15	1704	2556	2897	3238
15.5	1740	2610	2958	3306
16	1777	2666	3021	3376
16.5	1815	2722	3086	3448
17	1852	2778	3148	3519
17.5	1888	2832	3210	3587
18	1926	2889	3274	3659
18.5	1964	2946	3339	3732
19	2000	3000	3400	3800
19.5	2038	3057	3465	3872
20	2075	3112	3528	3942

For every additional stone increase daily calorie intake by 50

Notes

Chapter One: Living in a World Gone Mad: Fads, Fashions and Folly

1. *Daily Mail*, letters page, 24 January 2001.
2. The Size 8 Club Information Pack.
3. Reissued in 1994 as *The Forbidden Body: Why Being Fat Is Not a Sin*.
4. 'All Kinds of Everything', Leader Column, *Daily Telegraph*, 11 May 1998.
5. Nigella Lawson, 'Thin End of the Wedge', *Observer*, 14 January 2001.
6. Germaine Greer, 'Obscenity of the Finger Food Feasters', *Guardian*, 6 September 1993.
7. Joan Smith, 'Between the Beauty Myths', *Independent on Sunday*, 28 May 2001.
8. Llewellyn Louderback, *Fat Power*, Hawthorn Books, New York, 1970.
9. Christina Lamb, 'Eat, Eat, Eat', *Sunday Telegraph*, 25 March 2001.
10. Twiggy Lawson with Penelope Dening, Simon and Schuster, London, 1997.
11. Shelley Bovey, *The Forbidden Body*, Pandora, London, 1994.
12. *Journal of the American Medical Association*, March 2000.
13. Alison Dudley, Nicky Willshire, Joe Jeal, Andrea Valentine, 'We're All Size 10', *Daily Mail*, 11 July 2000.
14. Suzanne Moore, 'Refusing to Eat is Not a Disease, but a Solution to an Impossible Dilemma', *Guardian*, 24 October 1997.
15. The Size 8 Club Information Pack.
16. Liz Jones, 'I Expose the Guilty Fashion Editors who Drive Young Women to Starve Themselves', *Mail on Sunday*, 15 April 2001.
17. Courtney Thorne-Smith, 'My Life on the Ally McBeal Diet,' *Looks* Magazine, February 2001.
18. People, *The Week*, 5 May 2001.

19. Alison Boshoff, 'Uma Thurman, the Beauty who Sees a Fat Woman in her Mirror', *Daily Mail*, 21 February 2001.
20. Lowri Turner, 'Triumph for Largesse', *The Express*, 2 August 1998.
21. *Ibid.*
22. Andrew G Marshall, 'No One's Getting Fat Except Mama Cass', *Guardian*, 26 July 1999.
23. *Ibid.*
24. Board of Science, 'Eating Disorders, Body Image and the Media', The British Medical Association, May 2000.
25. Sandra Barwick, 'Thin Stars on TV "Put Pressure on the Young"', *Daily Telegraph*, 31 May 2000.
26. Nicci Gerrard, 'The Girl of my Dreams', *Observer*, 21 May 2000.
27. Liz Jones, 'I Expose the Guilty Fashion Editors who Drive Young Women to Starve Themselves', *Mail on Sunday*, 15 April 2001.
28. *Ibid.*
29. *Ibid.*
30. Sally Weale, 'Solidly Sexy and Totally in Vogue', *Guardian*, 17 May 1997.
31. *Ibid.*
32. 'Food for Thought', the Size 8 Club Information Pack.
33. Nigella Lawson, *Observer*, op. cit.
34. Aaron Lynch, *Thought Contagion*, Basic Books, New York, 1996, supported by author's article on the Internet: 'Thought Contagions and Pathological Dieting', based on an email and telephone interview with Megan McCafferty of *Glamour* magazine, February 2000.
35. *Ibid.*
36. Quoted by Suzanne Stevenson, 'Big "is Not Beautiful"', *Daily Mail*, 12 October 2000.
37. *Ibid.*
38. Web magazine, newwomen.co.uk, February 2001.
39. Suzanne Moore, *Guardian*, op. cit.
40. Nigella Lawson, 'Never Mind the Size, Just Feel the Price', *Observer*, 3 September 2000.
41. Nicci Gerrard, *Observer*, op.cit.
42. Joan Smith, *Independent on Sunday*, op.cit.

Chapter Two: Unlikely Bedfellows?: Reconciling Size Acceptance
and the Desire for Weight Loss
1. Personal communication.
2. State of the Movement Address, NAAFA newsletter,
    July/Aug 1997.
3. Shelley Bovey, *The Forbidden Body*, Pandora, London, 1994.
4. Jane Goddard Carter, 'Full Fat', in Shelley Bovey, ed, *Sizeable
    Reflections: Big Women Living Full Lives*, The Women's Press,
    London, 2000.
5. Charlotte Cooper, *Fat and Proud*, The Women's Press,
    London, 1998.
6. Maggie Millar, 'Correct Weight Is for Horses', paper given at
    a seminar on body image, for health professionals, Melbourne,
    9 May 1999.
7. *Freesize*, **2**.

Chapter Three: A Question of Identity
1. Made by Katherine Gilday, 1990.
2. *Ibid*.
3. *Ibid*.
4. Camryn Manheim, *Wake Up, I'm Fat*, Broadway Books, New
    York, 1999.
5. Shelley Bovey, *Being Fat Is Not a Sin*, Pandora, London,
    1989.
6. Susan Stinson, *Martha Moody*, The Women's Press, London,
    1996.
7. Bovey, op. cit.

Chapter Four: Why Do We Get Fat?
1. The Association for the Study of Obesity.
2. Personal communication, 12 May 2001.
3. *Ibid*.
4. Research quoted in Shelley Bovey, *The Forbidden Body*,
    Pandora, London, 1994.
5. Lisa Colles, *Fat: Exploding the Myths*, Carlton, London, 1998.
6. *Ibid*.
7. Eric Schlosser, *Fast Food Nation*, Houghton Mifflin, Boston,
    2001.
8. Shelley Bovey, *Being Fat Is Not a Sin* (now *The Forbidden Body*).
9. Personal communication, 12 May 2001.

Chapter Five: Seven Irrefutable, Unarguable Reasons Why You Should Not Lose Weight

1. GL Maddox and V Liederrnan, 'Overweight as a Social Disability with Medical Implications', *Journal of Medical Education* 44 (1969).
2. Thomas Stuttaford, 'How to Stop Diet Cheats', *The Times*, 7 June 2001.
3. Thomas Stuttaford, 'A Model for Weight Loss, *The Times*, 31 May 2001.
4. Shelley Bovey, *The Forbidden Body*, Pandora, London, 1994.
5. Charles Roy Schroeder, *Fat is Not a Four-Letter Word*, Chronimed Publishing, Minneaolis, 1992.
6. *Ibid.*
7. Lisa Colles, *Fat: Exploding the Myths*, Carlton, London, 1998.
8. HT Waaler, 'Height, Weight and Mortality: the Norwegian Experience', *acta med. Scand. Supp.* (1984) 679 1–56.
9. Paul Ernsserger and Paul Haskew, *Rethinking Obesity*, Human Sciences Press Inc, New York, 1987.
10. Broadway Books, New York, 1999.
11. Suzanne Moore, 'What Use Are the Celebrity Bodies with Empty Minds', *Mail on Sunday*, 8 April 2001.
12. Vanessa Feltz, 'Fattism', *Daily Mail*, 15 February 2001.
13. Karen Marchbank, quoted in 'Fat is a Careerist Issue', *Woman's Realm*, 27 February 2001.
14. *Ibid.*
15. BodyPositive.com.
16. Personal communication, 22 February 2001.

Chapter Six: A Personal Odyssey

1. Shelley Bovey, *Being Fat Is Not a Sin*, now issued as *The Forbidden Body: Why Being Fat Is Not a Sin*, Pandora, London, 1994.
2. Shelley Bovey, ed, *Sizeable Reflections – Big Women Living Full Lives*, The Women's Press, London, 2000.

Chapter Seven: How Not to Lose Weight

1. Paul Ernsberger and Paul Haskew, *Rethinking Obesity: An Alternative View of its Health Implications*, Human Sciences Press Inc, New York, 1987.

2. Shelley Bovey, *The Forbidden Body*, Pandora,London, 1994.
3. Gary Taubes, 'The Soft Science of Dietary Fat', *Science Magazine online*, 9 April 2001.
4. Meir Stampfer, Harvard professor of epidemiology and nutrition, quoted in Paul Kendall, 'Denying Yourself Fatty Food May Not Be Good for You', *Daily Mail*, 31 March 2001.
5. Barry Groves, *Eat Fat, Get Thin*, Vermilion, London, 1999.
6. Lois Rogers, 'Low-fat Diet May Pile on Weight', *The Sunday Times*, 4 January 1998.
7. *Ibid*.
8. Dr Jill Welbourne, personal communication.
9. Study quoted by Barry Groves, *op cit*.
10. Beckie King, MRC Human Nutrition Research, Personal communication, 4 July 2001.
11. Personal communication, 9 January 2001.
12. Barry Groves, *op. cit*.
13. 15 February 2001.
14. KR Westerterp, 'Pattern and Intensity of Physical Activity', *Nature*, **410**, 29 March 2001.
15. Belinda Charlton, *Big Is Invisible*, Robin Clark, London, 1985.
16. Editorial, *New Scientist*, 5 August 2000.
17. Ernsberger and Haskew, *op. cit*.
18. Anthony Harris, *The Catalogue of Diet Sheets*, Windward, Leicester, 1983.
19. Normandie Keith, 'Belly's Gonna Get Ya!' *You* magazine, 22 April 2001.
20. Dr Glenn Cooper and Tessa Cooper, *The Two-Day Diet*, Pan, London, 1988.
21. Martin Katahn, *The Rotation Diet*, Bantam Press, London, 1987.
22. Gene and Joyce Daoust, *The Formula*, Vermilion, London, 2001.
23. Clare Thompson, 'A Fat Lot of Good', *Sunday Times Magazine*, 23 February 1997.
24. John Humphrys, *Devil's Advocate*, Arrow, London, 1999.
25. *Ibid*.
26. Lisa Colles, *Fat: Exploding the Myths*, Carlton, London, 1998.
27. Ann Robinson, 'Last Chance to Be Slim, *Guardian*, 19 September 2000.
28. Keith Edington, Buckinghamshire County Council.

29. Lisa Colles, *Fat: Exploding the Myths*, Carlton, London, 1998.

Chapter Eight: Losing It: The Bad News
1. Barry Groves, *Eat Fat, Get Thin*, Vermilion, London, 1999.
2. Vanessa Feltz, 'Fattism', *Daily Mail*, 15 February 2001.
3. Suzanne Moore, 'Refusing to Eat is Not a Disease, but a Solution to an Impossible Dilemma', *Guardian*, 24 October 1997.

Chapter Nine: How to Lose Weight (and Keep Your Sanity)
1. www.caloriecontrol.org/exercalc.html.
2. Glenn Gaesser, *The Spark*, Simon and Schuster, New York, 2001.
3. Jane Goddard Carter, 'Full Fat', in Shelley Bovey, ed, *Sizeable Reflections: Big Women Living Full Lives*, The Women's Press, London, 2000.
4. Bull Publishing, Palo Alto, CA, 1990.
5. A Keys, et al, *The Biology of Human Starvation*, University of Minnesota Press, 1950.
6. Unable to believe this I checked with Jill Welbourne – the sufferer, Pauline Seaward, did indeed eat all that in one binge.
7. Rick Kausman, *If Not Dieting, Then What?*, Allen & Unwin, Australia, 1998.

Chapter Ten: Don't Go It Alone: The Importance of Support
1. Eg Susan Jebb of the Association for the Study of Obesity (ASO), personal communication, 8 January 2001.
2. *Ibid*.
3. Personal communication, 10 May 2001.
4. Personal communication, 3 February 2001.

Chapter Twelve: Keeping It Off For Ever
1. John Briffa, *Body Wise*, Cima Books, London, 2000.
2. Rick Kausman, *If Not Dieting, Then What?*, Allen & Unwin, Australia, 1998.
3. *Ibid*.
4. Lisa Colles, *Fat: Exploding the Myths*, Carlton, London, 1998.
5. *Ibid*, a generally agreed fact, quoted in this instance by nutritionist Rosemary Stanton in the foreword to this book.

Jill Welbourne made the same point, stating that for a person of 20 stone, losing just 2 stone would confer significant health benefits.

6. 'A Descriptive Study of Individuals Successful at Long-term Maintenance of Substantial Weight Loss', *American Journal of Clinical Nutrition*, 66, 2 (1997), 239–246.

7. Professor Stephen Bloom of the Hammersmith Hospital, in debate with the author, BBC Three Counties Radio, 30 July 2001.

Appendix:

1. WN Schofield, WPT James, 'Basal Metabolic Rate, Review and Prediction', *hum nutr clin nutr* (1985) **39** (Supplement) 1–96.

Bibliography

Atkins, RC, *Dr Atkins' New Diet Revolution*, Vermilion, London, 1992

Bovey, Shelley, ed, *Sizeable Reflections: Big Women Living Full Lives*, The Women's Press, London, 2000

Bovey, Shelley, *The Forbidden Body: Why Being Fat Is Not a Sin*, Pandora, London, 1994

Briffa, Dr J, *Bodywise*, Cima Books, London, 2000

Charlton, Belinda, *Big Is Invisible*, Robin Clark, London, 1985

Citron, J, *The Little Book of Slimming Tips*, Metro Books, London, 2000

Colles, L, *Fat: Exploding the Myths*, Carlton, London, 1998

Cooke, K, *Real Gorgeous*, Bloomsbury, London, 1994

Cooper, Charlotte, *Fat and Proud*, The Women's Press, London, 1998

Cooper, Dr Glen and Tessa Cooper, *The Two-Day Diet*, Pan, London, 1988

Daoust, G and Daoust, J, *The Formula*, Vermilion, London, 2001

Edison, LT and Notkin, D, *Women en Large: Images of Fat Nudes*, Books in Focus, San Francisco, 1994

Ernsberger, P and Haskew, P, *Rethinking Obesity: An Alternative View of its Health Implications*, Human Sciences Press, New York, 1987

Goodman, W Charisse, *The Invisible Woman: Confronting Weight Prejudice in America*, Gurze Books, California, 1995

Groves, Barry, *Eat Fat, Get Thin*, Vermilion, London, 1999

Harris, C, *Think Yourself Slim: A Unique Approach to Weight Loss*, Element, Shaftesbury, 1999

Jackson, S and Wallace, G, eds, *Women of Substance*, Allen and Unwin, Australia, 1998

Katahn, Martin, *The Rotation Diet*, Bantam Press, London, 1987

Kausman, Dr R, *If Not Dieting, Then What?*, Allen & Unwin, Australia, 1998

Klein, R, *Eat Fat*, Picador, London, 1996

Louderback, Llewellyn, *Fat Power: Whatever You Weigh is Right*, Hawthorn Books. New York, 1970

Lyons, P and Burgard, D, *Great Shape: The First Fitness Guide for Large Women*, Bull Publishing Company, California, 1990

Macdonald Baker, Dr S and Baar, K, *The Body Clock Diet*, Vermilion, London, 2000

Manheim, Camryn, *Wake Up, I'm Fat*, Broadway Books, New York, 1999

Schroeder, CR, *Fat Is Not a Four-Letter Word*, Chronimed Publishing, Minneapolis, 1992

Schwartz, H, *Never Satisfied: A Cultural History of Diets, Fantasies and Fat*, The Free Press, New York, 1986

Stinson, Susan, *Martha Moody*, The Women's Press, London, 1996

Tebbel, C, *The Body Snatchers: How the Media Shapes Women*, Finch Publishing, Sydney, 2000

Wann, M, *Fat!So?*, Ten Speed Press, California, 1998

Resources

Size Acceptance Organisations

National Association to Advance Fat Acceptance (NAAFA)
PO Box 188620
Sacramento
CA 95818, USA
Tel: 001916 558 6880
Fax: 001916 558 6881

The National Size Acceptance Network (SIZE)
Diana Pollard
10 Palace Gate
London W8 5NF

Health and Fitness at Any Size

Kathryn Szrodecki (Fitness classes for large women)
Alternative Size
1 Novello Street
London SW6 4JB
Tel: 020 7731 7436

Deb Burgard (co-author of *Great Shape*, the first fitness guide for
large women) www.bodypositive.com
('Boosting body image at any weight'.)

The Healthy Mind and Body Chart (a booklet and chart based on
maximising fitness: a vast improvement on the *BMI* chart)
Adelaide Nutrition Care
11 Bagot Street
North Adelaide
South Australia 5006
Email: nutritioncare@ozemail.com.au

Weight Loss Information and Support

The Obesity Research and Information Council (ORIC)
64 Great Eastern Street
London EC2A 3QR
Tel: 020 7613 7100
Fax: 020 7613 7101

The Obesity Solutions and Awareness Trust (TOAST)
The Latton Bush Centre
Southern Way
Harlow
Essex CM18 7BL
Tel/Fax: 01279 866010

Obesity Lifeline
Tel: 01279 306666
www.slimtime.co.uk
www.weightlossresources.co.uk

Slimming World
PO Box 55
Alfreton
Derbyshire DE55 4UE
Tel: 01773 520022
Fax: 01773 521880

Weight Watchers
Tel: 08457 123000

Rosemary Conley Diet and Fitness Clubs
Quorn House
Meeting Street
Quorn LE12 8EX
Tel: 01509 620222

General

Lee Kennedy cartoons
58 Durrington Tower
Wandsworth Road
London SW8 3LF
http://home.talkcity.com/PicassoPL/Droolcrone
http://homepages.msn.com/StageSt/Crazycrone/index.html

The Size 8 Club
14 Staple Hill
Wellesbourne
Warwickshire CV35 9LH
Tel: 01789 842307
Fax: 01789 842503
Email: helena.lomax@virgin.net

Soehnle Scales
Austin White (Northampton) Ltd
Unit 2, 3 Mansard Close
Westgate Interstate Estate
Northampton NN5 5DL
Tel: 01604 588992
Fax: 01604 588803

Verity (an organisation for Polycystic-ovary Syndrome sufferers)
52–54 Featherstone Street
London EC1Y 8RT
www.verity-pcos.org.uk